EDUCATION IN A COMPETITIVE AND GLOBALIZING WORLD

SELECTED TOPICS ON PRE-K-6 HEALTH EDUCATION

FROM RESEARCH TO PRACTICE

EDUCATION IN A COMPETITIVE AND GLOBALIZING WORLD

Additional books in this series can be found on Nova's website under the Series tab.

Additional e-books in this series can be found on Nova's website under the e-book tab.

EDUCATION IN A COMPETITIVE AND GLOBALIZING WORLD

SELECTED TOPICS ON PRE-K-6 HEALTH EDUCATION

FROM RESEARCH TO PRACTICE

CECILIA OBENG, PH.D.
Department of Applied Health Science
Indiana University

NOVINKA

New York

For permission to use material from this book please contact us:
Telephone 631-231-7269; Fax 631-231-8175
Web Site: http://www.novapublishers.com

Library of Congress Cataloging-in-Publication Data

ISBN: 978-1-63321-754-6

Published by Nova Science Publishers, Inc. † New York

This book is dedicated to my mother Margaret Aboagyewaa,
and my stepmother, Hannah Korankyewaa
who made the most impact in my early childhood.

CONTENTS

PREFACE

This book discusses health education for children, particularly for preschool and elementary age children. This area of health education among children is very important because of a recent increase in childhood health problems (Ogden Yanovski, Carroll, Flegal (2007)).

The above problems motivated the author to write this book. All chapters are based on research from experiences with parents, and teachers in childcare/preschool, elementary schools, and on the author's personal experience as a practitioner.

The early years are the most important years in a child's life and because of that, preschool health education should not focus on teachers and children only, but should also help parents as well. Based on the scholarly work in the area of health education in the early years, the following recommendations are made.

Although teachers see health activities as important, some teachers are focusing on personal health only. Educators can do better if they cover physical activity, nutrition, emotional health issues, and other health-related topics in their classrooms. Teachers can integrate physical activities in every facet of children's classrooms to help curb childhood health problems.

Cecilia S. Obeng, Ph.D.
Indiana University- School of Public Health
1025 E. 7th Street
SPH 116 Bloomington, Indiana, US 47405
Tel: 812-856-0502
cobeng@indiana.edu

REFERENCES

Ogden, C. L., Yanovski, S. Z., Carroll, M. D., & Flegal, K. M. (2007). The Epidemiology of Obesity, *Gastroenterology, 132*(6), 2087-3010.

ACKNOWLEDGMENTS

The writing of this book would not have been possible without the help of Professor Samuel Obeng (my husband). Dr. Tristan Purvis read through earlier drafts of the manuscript and made useful suggestions and I am very thankful to him. Jessica Hauser read through the final version of the book and I am very grateful to her. Finally, I am grateful to my children, Samilia, Emmanuel, and Barnabas, for their encouragement.

Chapter 1

PARENTS' FEELINGS ON UNDER-AGED CHILDREN'S ASSOCIATION WITH, AND CONSUMPTION OF ALCOHOL

ABSTRACT

This chapter examines how parents express valence about children's association with alcohol-use via specific kinds of vocabulary items and expressions made up of adjectives and intensifiers, and word repetition. The study took place in Accra, Ghana, and involved transcripts of data collected from seventy-eight (78) participants. Working within the frameworks of *valence* (Frijda, 1986; Lerner and Keltner, 2000) and the *(bad) news delivery* (Maynard, 1997), the study shows that negative valence (especially, sorrow and anger) about children's possible alcohol-use was expressed with specific *intensifiers*, *moral-induced words*, and *word repetition*. There was difference in how male and female respondents expressed valence about introducing alcohol to children in early years. Given the gender differences in expressing feelings about probable alcohol-use among children, it is recommended that stakeholders pay attention to such communicative differences to ensure that such education reaches both genders.

INTRODUCTION

Children and Alcohol Use

The works of Koriah (2003) and Obeng (2011) indicate the cultural acceptance of early alcohol use due, in part, to alcoholic drinks being used at children's naming ceremonies, festivals, and funerals. The authors also explicate the ease with which children can obtain and use alcohol in African societies and the risks associated with easy access to alcohol.

Language and Gender

With respect to the interconnectedness between language and gender, the works of West and Zimmermann (1983), Romine (1994), Talbot (2010), and many others indicate differences in male and female speech. West and Zimmermann (1983) for example note that in an average conversation, women ask 70% of the questions, and men interrupt 96% of the time. A more recent work on language and gender is that of Talbot (2010) in which she provides a thorough argument about the significance of language and gender in the synthesis and analysis of popular culture, mass media texts, and sexuality.

Work on language and gender in medical discourse (West, 1984; 1990) shows that in patient-physician meetings, doctors tend to interrupt their patients male and female by two-to-one except when the doctor is a woman. Male patients, West (ibid) discovered, tend to interrupt female doctors more than female patients.

An important study relevant to our study is that by Holmes (1995) where she notes that men and women use language to achieve different communicative ends. Holmes notes that women pay more attention to the feelings of other interactional participants than men whereas men pay more attention to the content and outcome of talk. Thus, whereas women use language to establish, nurture and develop personal relationships men "tend to see language more as a tool for obtaining and conveying information. Men see talk as a means to an end, and the end can often be very precisely defined — a decision reached, for instance, some information gained, or a problem resolved" (Holmes, 1995:2).

As far as we know, there is no study on language and gender in the expression of valence about children's association with alcohol use. This study, therefore, aims at filling that gap by examining how Ghanaian parents express valence about probable alcohol use by children

DATA AND METHOD

Data

The data for the study consisted of transcripts of completed questionnaires administered in Ghana between November and December of 2009. Human subject authorization endorsement was sought from Indiana University's Human Subjects Committee prior to the commencement of the data gathering. The research participants were parents of school-aged children. Research participants were contacted through teachers and school administrators. The teachers and school administrators made arrangements for the researchers to meet with the research participants who had time and were willing to meet. Participants who had e-mails were contacted via e-mails. Of the 104 parents who completed the research questions, 78 (72.9%) answered the questions that formed the basis of this study.

Study Instrument

The main study's data collection instrument contained closed- and open-ended questions. The questions were designed to ensure participants' anonymity. The instrument for the current study focused on the important issues of *how participants would feel if they saw a child consuming alcohol*; The original research questions were pilot tested to ensure their cultural aptness, then revised taking into account problems that arose from the pilot study (see Obeng, 2011), and then administered in this study.

Procedure

The author and two, paid research assistants collected the data. The questionnaires were distributed to research participants by hand and via e-mail. Research participants completed the research questionnaire on their own free time and free will and the completed answers were collected either in person or via e-mail.

Theoretical Underpinnings

This study is done within the frameworks of *valence* (Lerner and Keltner, 2000; Frijda, 1986) and *(bad) news delivery* Maynard (2003). Working within the framework of valence (Frijda, 1986; Lerner and Keltner, 2000) enabled us to determine how research participants' negative feelings about children's association with alcohol influenced their choice of words to index how they felt. It also enabled us to scrutinize the words they used to express and/or state what they believed should happen to those who introduced children to alcohol.

Following Maynard's (2003) work on *good/bad news delivery*, allowed us to explore how participants expressed negative/bad valence through the use of specific vocabulary and expressions. In particular, Maynard's model provided us with a window of opportunity to examine, through language, how participants anticipated or came to realize their children's potential 'new' world (that of potentially becoming alcoholic) and the probable attendant consequences of alcoholism.

Results

Common Themes

Common themes that emerged across the data included:

(a) What alcohol can do; that is, the destructive effects of alcohol on children's thinking-process and on their behavior;
(b) Alcohol's capacity to destroy and cause disease in the human physiology, especially in the functioning of such vital organs as the brain, heart, liver, and kidney; and
(c) Issues on morality whereby the research participants saw alcohol use as immoral and hence the need to prevent alcoholism and teach good morals.

How Men Would Feel If Children Used Alcohol

In expressing their feelings about children's association and probable use of alcohol, male research participants used such emotion-laden adjectives as *afraid, bad, disappointed, scared, sad, sorry, surprised, uncertain, uncomfortable, uneasy,* and *worried* to index valence. The word *very* (which is an *intensifier*) and its reduplicated version "*very, very*" were used to emphasize and thus show via the degree of intensity of the adjectives, the extent of valence — *disappointment, discomfort, fear, sadness,* or *uncertainty* — towards children's association with alcohol. In the English language, intensifiers, by nature, have a heightening or lowering effect on meaning (Crystal, 1985) so their use in expressing the extent of valence served as a reinforcement of the degree of the research participants' rejection of alcohol use by children. Examples of excerpts explicating their negative valence include:

A: bad, scared for the next generation
B: very, very bad
C: feel bad
D: I will feel bad, because taking alcohol can kill you
E: sad and would advise him
F: sad
G: very sad
H: disappointed and bad
I: very uneasy
J: very uneasy, do not drink
K: very, very uncomfortable
L: surprised
M: afraid and worried for his/her future
N: beat my child
O: that particular child is in trouble as in drinking [sic]; well his/her future is at stake

Purported action that the participants vowed to take to correct the potential wrong or immoral act pointed to the extent of valence. Such actions included: *going after the one who offered the alcohol to the child; issuing a stern warning to such children, advising the children, and in extreme cases resolving to use physical or corporal punishment if need be.* For example, a research participant noted: *I will beat my child.*

An observation to the data showed that in expressing the action they would take, the first person pronoun, *I,* was used to denote or symbolize authority on the part of the respondents and to amplify their power to socialize, and more specifically, to straighten up their children to ensure that they abstain from alcohol. Use of the first person singular pronoun appears to suggest something like: "I, who am the parent and therefore have the power to take action..."

With respect to why they felt the way they indicated, respondents noted that their feelings were motivated by the capacity of alcohol to kill and destroy individuals and to the fact that the future of their children was at stake when it came to alcohol consumption due to alcohol's lasting impact on an individual's health. Examples of excerpts include:

A: I will feel bad, because taking alcohol can kill you.
B: Afraid and worried for his/her future; and
C: That particular child is in trouble as in drinking [sic], well his/her future is at stake

How Women Would Feel If Children Used Alcohol

Female respondents used emotion-laden adjectives and expressions such as; heartbroken, worried, sad, pathetic, disappointed and sorry, sad and pity, bad and worried, sad and worried, scared for his future, not happy, unhappy, and disturbed to describe the nature and extent of valence. As can be scrutinized from the entire data, men used one adjective at a time to express valence, whereas women used more than one adjective in every single situation. Also, women used more intensifiers than men (2 to 1 ratio) to emphasize the degree of intensity or strength inherent in the adjective to show the extent of valence. The intensifiers used by the female respondents included; so, very, very, very, and very much.

Purported action expressed as part of our consequence of valence included: readiness to take suitable action to halt such deviant and irresponsible behavior; educating the public, victims and adult offenders; dismissal of offenders from employment; and if it is determined that nothing humanly possible could be done, then hoping for divine intervention.

Given that the above adjectives and intensifiers index valence, it could be argued that women's use of more adjectives and intensifiers than men point to the higher level of their expression of valence. This may be motivated by gender roles in Ghanaian society that lays the burden of nurturing more on women than on men (see Obeng, 2011).

Regarding the reason(s) why the female respondents felt the way they did, the respondents noted that their feelings were motivated by: their knowledge of alcohol's power to destroy children's lives, their health, and their future; the fact that it is morally wrong for children to engage in drinking; the fact that alcoholism leads to death; and the fact that some parents may not be aware of what their children are engaged in.

Discussion and Conclusion

This study has shown that parents' objection to children's association with alcohol-use can be gleaned from the strength of the language they use to express valence — be it anger, sadness, or sorrow. Use of such emotional valence-laden language helps to amplify the extent of the social problem parents are faced with and sheds light on how they want such a problem to be tackled or solved.

This study's research participants' determination to seek help (divine or human) in order to ensure their children's safety, and the reasons they give as motivation for such support, go a long way to show the extent to which parents in particular, and caregivers in general, will go to protect and safeguard children.

There is no doubt that in the studied area there were cultural factors that motivated the sending of children to purchase alcohol for adults and the early initiation of children to alcohol use; however, the sentiments expressed by parents against alcohol-use by children go a long way to emphasize the need to include their views in any policy on their children's welfare.

On the interconnectedness between language and gender and the expression of valence about alcohol use, this study has shown that even though there are similarities in ways in which males and females express abhorrence, sadness, and empathy about a social problem, there are also unique ways associated with each gender group. This language and gender difference has significance for health communication. Specifically, it points to the fact that any public health education policy that ignores these communicative differences is bound to reach only a part of the population. In effect, this study supports and extends the works of Wierzbicka (1991) and Holmes (1995) which call for close and systematic attention to gender differences in communication and for the need to pay attention to both genders in the production and dissemination of educational information.

Furthermore, this study supports Maynard's (1997) study on *bad news delivery* that calls for attention to be paid to ways of expressing valence (especially, bad news) since such knowledge helps us to understand what is being said by interlocutors as well as the interlocutors' innermost feelings about the subject matter of what is said. Thus, this study amplifies Maynard's position about the extent to which interlocutors' words index and are signaled by their emotion and empathy with the people about whom they speak. An understanding about interlocutors' innermost feelings has the potential to assist us in placing ourselves in the same camera-angle as them and subsequently to enable us to come up with solutions that are acceptable to them and to other stakeholders.

Finally, working within Maynard's model has allowed us to show the implications of our study for understanding a social problem, that of alcoholism. Specifically, working on the conveyance of valence in the form of 'bad news' has provided us with etic-based knowledge that will enable us to make recommendations for stakeholders (parents, policy makers, and professional educators), on how to come up with ways for effectively carrying out a public health education program — that of abstention from potential alcohol abuse.

REFERENCES

American Association for Marriage and Family Therapy. (2010). http://www.aamft.org/families/consumer_updates/substanceabuseandintimaterelationships.as_Accessed November 24, 2010.

Centers for Disease Control and Prevention. (2010). *Youth Risk Behavior Survey* (YRBS). Available at: http://www.cdc.gov/features/riskbehavior/. Accessed November 1, 2010.

Crystal, D. (1985). *A dictionary of linguistics and phonetics*. New York: Basil Blackwell.

DeWit, D. J., Adlaf, E. M., & Offord, D. R. (2000). Age at First Alcohol Use: A risk factor for the development of alcohol disorders. *American Journal of Psychiatry 157*(5), 745–750.

Frijda, N. H. (1986). *The Emotions*. Cambridge (UK): Cambridge University Press.

Holmes, J. (1995) *Women, Men and Politeness.* London and New York: Longman

Koriah C. J. (2006). Alcohol and empire: "illicit" gin prohibition and control in colonial Eastern Nigeria. *African Economic History 31*, 111-134.

Hingson, R.W.; Heeren, T.; & Winter, M. R. (2006). Age at drinking onset and alcohol dependence: age at onset, duration, and severity. *Archives of Pediatrics & Adolescent Medicine* 160(7), 739-746.

Lerner, J. S. & Keltner, Dacher (2000). Beyond valence: Toward a model of emotion-specific influences on judgment and choice. *Cognition & Emotion* 14(4), 473-493.

Maynard, D. (2003). *Bad News, Good News: Conversational Order in Everyday Talk and Clinical Settings*. Chicago: The University of Chicago Press

Obeng, C. S. (2011). Parental Perspectives on Alcohol Use among School–Aged Children in Ghana. *The International Electronic Journal of Health Education*

Romaine, S. (1994). *Language in Society; An Introduction to Sociolinguistics.* Oxford University Press.

Talbot, M. M. (2010). *Language and Gender.* Cambridge (UK): Polity Press.

West, C. (1984). Routine complications: troubles with talk between doctors and patients. Bloomington: Indiana University Press.

West, C. & Zimmerman, D. H. (1983). Small insults: A study of interruptions in cross-sex conversations between unacquainted persons. In B. Thorne, C. Kramarae, & N. Henley (Eds.) *Language, gender and society.* Cambridge, MA: Newbury House.

Wierzbicka, A. (1991) *Cross-Cultural Pragmatics: the Semantics of Human Interaction*. Berlin: Mouton de Gruyter.

Young, S. Y., Hansen, C. J., & Gibson R. L. (2006). Risky alcohol use, age at onset of drinking, and adverse childhood experiences in young men entering the US Marine Corps. *Archives of Pediatrics & Adolescent Medicine* 160(12): 1207-1214.

Chapter 2

IMMIGRANT CHILDREN'S SCHOOLING IN THE UNITED STATES

BACKGROUND TO CHAPTER

This chapter explores school attendance among African immigrant school-aged children by examining illnesses that their parents consider prevalent, 'serious,' or 'ordinary' and how such perceptions influence their decision to allow their children to attend or miss school.

The data for the study were collected in Indiana and Virginia between 2005 and 2008 by the author and three research assistants. A total of one hundred and five families took part in the research, answering closed- and open-ended questions about their children.

More than half of the immigrant parents surveyed in the study ensured that their children's illness did not interrupt their school attendance. Most participants scheduled their children's doctor's appointments during non-school hours. Missing school was viewed as being a failure or inability on the part of a parent to properly socialize their child to enjoy hard work. Some participants viewed missing school as not taking advantage of the opportunity they have in their new environment (USA). The study concludes that the immigrants' cultures have considerable impact on their perceptions about health and school attendance. The study could form the basis for studying the link between health and schooling among different immigrant groups.

INTRODUCTION

There is a dearth of knowledge on the close connection between health and school attendance among children the world over. The little that has been done has been completed in some American populations with recent immigrant populations often ignored. In their study of symptom profile and asthma control among urban minority school-aged children, Vargas et al. (2006) show that children with poorly controlled asthma are at high risk of school absenteeism, limited participation in activities, and in sleep disruption. Furthermore, the authors discovered the prevalence of poor asthma control among the children—a situation that they identified as being responsible for the poor school attendance and inferior quality of life of the children (see also, Levi et al. (2006)).

An important aspect of health and school attendance deals with parental perception of the severity of their child's illness. In their study of social context influencing pain and pain behavior, Goubert et al. (2006) saw that parents' thinking about the acuteness of their child's pain significantly contributed their children's school attendance as well as parental depression and anxiety.

With respect to the positive impact of health improvement on school attendance, Mahawithange et al.'s (2007) study of the impact of Vitamin A supplementation on health status and absenteeism of schoolchildren, showed that, if properly managed, Vitamin A supplementation with an appropriate IU dosage (200,000 IU) over an appropriate time period (every 4 months over 13 months) has a strong potential of improving vitamin A status and school attendance of the children.

Finally, in their work on anemia and school participation, Bobonis, Miguel, and Puri-Sharma (2006) demonstrated that such health intervention strategies as delivering iron supplementation and de-worming drugs to preschool children leads to an increase in preschool participation, reduction in absenteeism, and a curb in weight loss among the assisted children. The authors concluded that school-based health programs constitute an effective way of promoting school attendance.

Given the connection between health and school attendance as espoused in the above literature, and in view of the dearth of knowledge about health and school attendance among school-aged immigrant populations, the present study investigates:

(a) Illnesses that recent African immigrant parents believe are common among their school-aged children,
(b) The parents' perceptions about the illnesses, and
(c) How such perceptions influence their children's school attendance.

SITE AND DATA

The sites for this study were Virginia and Indiana. All participants from Indiana lived in Indianapolis and surrounding towns (fifty miles away from Indianapolis). The other participants lived in North Virginia, which is close to Washington D.C., the capital of the United States of America. The data were collected from 2005 to 2008 and were collected from professionals like nurses, teachers, and lawyers and from nonprofessionals like cab drivers, janitors, fast food workers, and students. In all, four people were involved in the data collection— the author and three graduate research assistants. One graduate research assistant did the survey at Virginia and the other two graduate assistants worked at Indiana. The personal interviews were conducted by the principal investigator and one graduate assistant. All the data collection was done in English and took place after an approval from an institutional review board.

Subject Selection

Participants were selected for this study through the snowball and purposeful sampling techniques (Patton, 1990). No incentives were provided to participants. Eligibility requirements included being an African immigrant parent with a child or children in school—preschool and school-aged children.

Procedure

After participants were identified, they were approached by either the author or her graduate assistants through e-mails, personal interactions, and phone-calls. Consent forms were given to participants to read. Of the one hundred and five participants, sixty-six filled in the questionnaire with pen/pencils by themselves, fourteen participants had theirs filled in by either the author or her research assistants, and the remaining twenty-five were tape-recorded by the principal investigator and one of the graduate research assistants who did face-to-face interviews with the participants. Questions were administered in participants' homes.

Research Questions

The research questions that guided this study elicited information on participants' native countries of origin, how long they had been in the United States, the number of children that they had, the most common illness(es) that their child or children had, and the influence of their children's illness on their school attendance.

Data Coding

Three people were involved in the coding process: the author, a colleague, and a graduate research assistant. The coding was done using the *constant comparative/constant comparison method*. The data were first coded by the author and the doctoral research assistant into four broad themes. The author and a colleague then took portions of the data and compared the themes identified to determine their relevance and similarity (Schwandt, 2001). This process was done until all important categories were under specific themes. The coders read the data and the themes that were identified separately. After reading the data they compared all the comments to make sure each segment put under any of the themes "qualified" to be under that theme. Their comments were discussed until all themes and the segments under them were agreed upon (Lewis-Beck, Bryman, and Liao, 2004).

Data Analysis

The analysis done for this study involves quoting of raw data from the research participants' utterances to support the analytical claims that are made. This type of analysis helps to inform readers about the research participants' perceptions regarding their health, and schooling, and it gives readers the knowledge about how the research participants viewed the health and education of their children in their own cultures. Since the analytical claims are based on participants' words, the conclusions drawn from the data, therefore, come from the participants themselves. Thus, any conclusions that are drawn help to amplify participants' voices instead of making them appear faceless in the study.

Findings

The findings of the paper address the following important issues: common illnesses of participants' children (including the participants' perception of what constitutes a serious illness and what motivates them to take their children to the clinic or hospital), and parents' reported time of taking their children to the clinic/hospital.

Demographic Information

Of the one hundred and five participants who took part in this study, 70.5% (N=74) were African immigrants from West African countries. The remaining 29.5% (N=31) were from other parts of Africa. These participants answered questions on 240 children. A majority of the participants had three kids (see Table 1 below).

Table 1. Participants' Demographics

Participants & Their Children	# Parent Participants	Total # Children
Participants with 1 Child	33	33
Participants with 2 Children	21	42
Participants with 3 Children	39	117
Participants with 4 Children	12	48
Total	105	240

Common Illnesses

The common illnesses reported by participants are cold and flu, ear infection, bacterial infection, fever, nausea, and nose bleeding. These are represented in Figure 1 below.

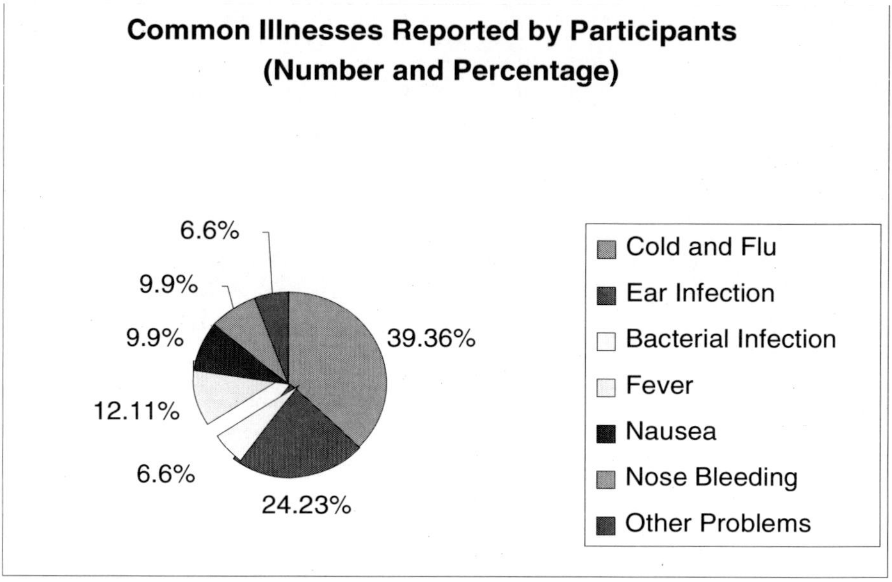

Figure 1. Common illness.

From the above figure, we learn that 39% of the surveyed parents indicated that the most common form of illness found in their children was cold and/or flu. They noted that at times their children had a cold for between six and eight times per year. Some parents reported that there were times that their child's cold or flu got so bad that they did not know what to do especially at night when their children struggled to breathe.

A participant noted:

> At times nobody in my house would sleep for even an hour or so. My son struggled to breathe most of the time. He never finished one-fourth of his food the day before, so I could see that he was very hungry. My husband and my younger brother would try to persuade him to eat but were not successful. Any time that he started coughing or I saw fluid coming from the nose, I knew another sleepless night awaited us. What we didn't want was for the school nurse to call us and to ask us to pick up our child from school because he was ill. It portrays us as being irresponsible. We therefore made sure he ate well and took his medicine.

Close observation of the data also shows that 24% of the participants' children had symptoms of ear infection after their cold.

A father noted:

> Once I know that her cold/flu goes beyond a week or more, then, I definitely knew the next thing she would complain about would be earache. I had to prepare my mind and work more hours to get money for her to see the doctor since there was no way an over-the-counter medicine would make her well. We were very careful not to let her have the illness for a long time without seeing the doctor since someone else in the family could also catch it. When so many people live together, you can support one another in times of illness and that is exactly what we did

Nine percent mentioned nausea and nose bleeding as the common illness that affected their children whereas 6% of the surveyed participants reported bacterial infection as being the common illness found in their children.

A man who had lived in the U.S. for three years wrote:

> He (referring to his son) had never had any problem with nose bleeding when we were at home [country of origin] but since our coming into this country, every year at least his nose bleeds twice or more. I always make sure he will not engage himself in any activity that will trigger his nose bleeding.

Twenty-four percent of the surveyed parents reported that the illness that led their school-aged children to see the doctor was ear infection although cold/flu was the illness reported most by participants.

Some parents from West Africa reported that in their culture the illness that they considered most serious was malaria. None of the parents reported that any of their children had such an illness in their new environment (the United States). For such parents, apart from malaria and yellow fever, no other disease should constitute the basis for their child missing school.

Other African immigrants, especially from southern Africa, reported viral and bacterial infections as being illnesses that they were afraid of. For such immigrants, if their child contracted a viral and/or bacterial infection, then the child might miss school.

The above observations are rooted in the participants' cultures and worldview in the sense that malaria is prevalent in West Africa whereas HIV and AIDS are common in southern Africa. The above findings also indicate that even in their new environment the immigrants' mindset about illness is shaped by the diseases in their home countries and that they are somehow still 'afraid' of the diseases that affect people in their native countries.

Time of Clinic/Hospital Attendance

From the data we observe that a majority of the participants (about 54.3%) reported that they set their children's hospital/clinic appointments after three o'clock—that is, after the school hours. A little over thirty-one percent (31.4%) of respondents set their children's appointments between 9:00 a.m. and 12:00 p.m. (noon), whereas 14.3% set theirs at between 12:00 p.m. (noon) and 3:00 p.m. (see Figure 2).

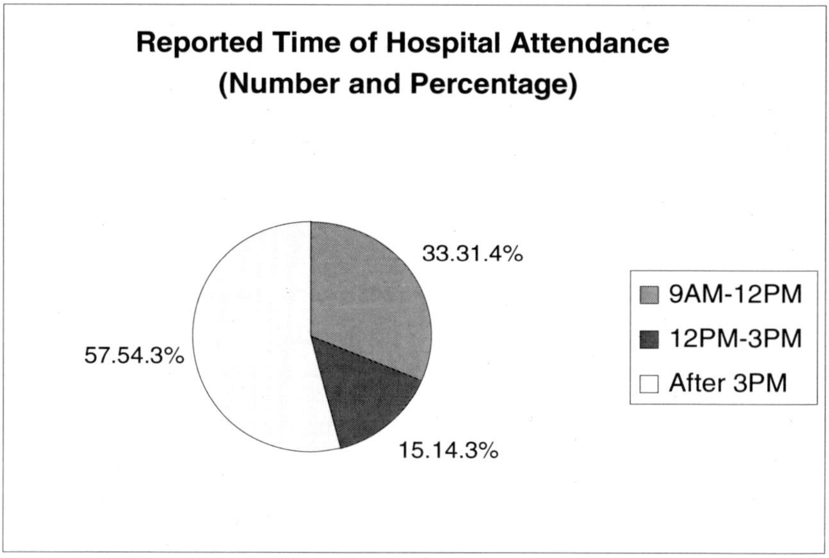

Figure 2. Time of Hospital Attendance.

The reason given by the surveyed participants for setting this particular time for their child to see the doctor was that if a child was not in serious pain or had no communicable illness, then there was no need to let the child miss school.

A participant who made every effort for his child not to miss school commented:

> I know my child has these multiple problems but I make sure she takes her medicine every evening before she goes to bed. I also make sure she gets enough sleep every day to be able to go to school. I'm from a family where my parents did not get any formal education but tried their best with their scarce resources to educate us (their eight children in total). I have every

> opportunity to help my children here in the United States since there are better facilities to support people.

From participants' utterances, we learn that their choice of time was motivated by their desire for their children not to miss any schoolwork in order for them to do well.

A female participant wrote:

> In my culture going to school is like working. You do not want to miss so many hours of work in order to get a good paycheck. The same applies to school. I do not want my child to miss so many hours of school because missing so many hours of schooling will definitely affect her grades. There are a lot of opportunities in this country; opportunities you don't find back home so missing school is like missing a great opportunity to do well in life.

DISCUSSION

Based on the findings discussed in the previous section, it may be argued that, for the surveyed parents, the prevalence of flu and cold were problematic to them cognizant of the fact that in their native countries such illnesses were uncommon. The parents found the prevalence of cold and flu among their children problematic given the impact of these illnesses on their children's schooling. In particular, the possibility of a school nurse summoning them to the school to pick up a child because of cold or flu was a situation they found difficult to comprehend and/or bear.

Also, given the fact that some of these immigrants lived with extended family members, the prevalence of cold and flu was not only problematic to the children's parents, but to everybody in the family—both nuclear and extended—since they all had to deal with it collectively by supporting one another.

Furthermore, a close attention to the data and to the findings point to the fact that the surveyed participants' view of the United States as a land of opportunity had considerable impact on their decision about the appropriate time for their children to see a physician as well as their decision to make a child miss school due to an illness. For most of the research participants, missing school meant not having a good grade and hence their decision to encourage a child who, in their opinion, was not very ill, to go to school. As one parent said, "*Missing school is like missing work.*" Thus, for them, missing school was like missing a paycheck, a rare but important lifetime opportunity.

Finally, through the utterances of the research participants, the study has shown the various illnesses that are common among the surveyed immigrant participants' children.

The study has also shown the surveyed participants' perceptions about the impact of such illnesses and/or diseases on their children's school attendance in particular, and the value the immigrant parents place on their children's schooling in general.

CONCLUSION

This study is of significance to health educators, medical practitioners, and social workers, as well as to teachers who deal with immigrant children. In particular, the findings of the study constitute a source of knowledge from which the above-mentioned professionals can learn about the impact of culture on health and school attendance among immigrant populations. Knowing about the parents' perceptions about illnesses and how their cultures influence the decisions they make during a child's sickness will help the professionals take appropriate and informed decisions. Thus, based on such knowledge, the professionals can make appropriate recommendations to the parents and the other stakeholders on the immigrant children's welfare for the betterment of the children's lives. This study could also form the basis for studying the link between culture, health, and schooling among other immigrant groups.

REFERENCES

Bobonis, G. J., Miguel, E., and Puri-Sharma, C. (2006). Anemia and school participation. *Journal of Human Resources*. 41(4): 692-721.

Goubert, L., Eccleston, C., Vervoort, T., Jordan, A., & Crombez, G. (2006). Parental catastrophizing about their child's pain. The parent version of the Pain Catastrophizing Scale (PCS-P): a preliminary validation. *Pain, 123*(3), 254-263.

Levi, M., Heffner, B., Stewart, T., & Beeman, G. (2006). The efficacy of asthma case management in an urban school district in reducing school absences and hospitalizations for asthma. *Journal of School Health, 76*(6), 320-324.

Lewis-Beck, M. S., Bryman, A., & Liao, T. F. (2004) *Encyclopedia of Social Science Research Methods Vol 2.* Thousand Oaks, CA: SAGE

Mahawithange, S. T. C., Kannanga, K. K. N. P., & Wickremasinghe, R. (2007). Impact of vitamin A supplementation on health status and absenteeism of school children in Sri Lanka. *Asia Pacific Journal of Clinical Nutrition, 16*(1), 94-102.

Patton, M. Q. (1990). *Qualitative Evaluation and Research Methods.* 2nd ed. Newbury Park, CA: Sage Publications.

Schwandt, T. A. (2001). *Dictionary of Qualitative Inquiry.* 2nd ed. Thousand Oaks, CA: Sage.

Vargas, P. A., Simpson, P. M., & Bushmiaer, M. (2006). Symptom profile and asthma control in school-aged children. *Annual Allergy Asthma Immunology 96*(6), 787-793.

Chapter 3

HEALTH LESSONS IN EARLY ELEMENTARY CLASSROOMS

ABSTRACT

Despite the fact that injuries are the leading cause of childhood deaths in industrialized countries (Kendrick et al., 2007), an observation of the literature on Health Education shows that very little research has been done on injury topics taught in kindergarten classrooms and why teachers teach them. This study examines injury prevention lessons taught in kindergarten classrooms and why the teachers taught them. The study employs *mixed methods.* Results indicate that a majority of the teachers taught *fire* and *playground safety*, whereas *gun safety* was taught by only a few. Some participants recommended involving safety personnel in teaching about safety.

INTRODUCTION

The need for children to understand the contributions that they can make towards injury prevention should be emphasized in their classrooms. This is because scholarship on childhood injury points to the fact that injuries are the leading cause of childhood deaths in industrialized countries (Kendrick et al., 2007).

With respect to the causes of injury sustained by children, Pickett, Ardern, and Brison's (2001) work indicates that *falls* are known to account for most cases of head injuries with boys having the tendency to sustain head injuries more than girls. Furthermore, girls are known to have lower risk for fatal injuries than boys.

Another important aspect of injury causation discussed in the literature is the extent to which area-level socioeconomic position influences the risk for childhood fatal injuries. For example, Kim, Subramanian, Kawachi, and Kim (2007) have discovered that children who reside in more deprived districts or non-metropolitan regions and rural areas are significantly associated with increased risk of injury.

An observation of the literature on injury indicates further that the incidence of injury increases with age (Dal Santo, Goodman, & Jackson, 2004) and that the incidence of injury among preschool children is lower than that of children ten years old and beyond.

With respect to the connection between parents' occupation type and children's injury, research has shown that children with fathers in manual occupations have higher risk of injuries than children whose fathers are in non-manual occupations (Kim, Subramanian, Kawachi, & Kim, 2007). Also, concerning the relationship between children's injuries and their parents' level of education, Kim, Subramanian, Kawachi and Kim (2007) have indicated that children with mothers whose highest level of education is high school or junior high school have a higher risk of getting injured than those whose mothers are college graduates.

Concerning physical activity and injury causation, Spinks, McClure, Bain, and Macpherson (2006) assert that, in spite of the fact that regular physical activity is strongly recommended for children, physical activity, if not properly supervised by adults, could expose children to the risks of injury. Scholars such as Schwebel, Brezausek, and Belsky (2006) have also worked on the extent to which the quantity and quality of early childcare influence children's risk for unintentional injury. Specifically, in their study of *the relationship between time spent in childcare and the risk for unintentional injury,* the authors discovered that children who spent more time in non-parental childcare environments were at slightly reduced risk for unintentional injury.

With respect to the impact of children's health knowledge and incidence of health risk, Knoff's (2001) work indicates that children's health risk decreases if they are introduced to appropriate health knowledge and skill at a younger age. The above claim gives credence to the need for teachers to assist children to establish injury prevention habits at a younger age. In seeking to understand the nature of topics on injury taught to children and why kindergarten teachers teach or do not teach injury topics, two main research questions are explored:

(a) What kind of injury topics do kindergarten teachers teach? and
(b) Why do the teachers teach certain topics but not others?

METHODOLOGY

The study employs both qualitative and quantitative research methods. For the qualitative method, an aspect of the *constant comparison* method (that of identifying recurrent themes) was used. Using constant comparison method enabled me to compare participants' ideas and to categorize such ideas into themes (Strauss & Corbin, 1998; Dye, Schatz, Rosenberg, & Coleman, 2000). For the quantitative aspect of this study, an association between binary categorical variables of interest was examined using chi-square test (df=1).

Population Sample

The population for the study was 120 kindergarten school teachers teaching in two Midwestern counties. This study was part of a bigger study about teachers who teach elementary-aged children. Out of 236 questionnaires completed by elementary school teachers (K-6), 120 were completed by kindergarten teachers. Only kindergarten school teachers were selected for this study because they were the group of teachers we chose them because we wanted to focus on teachers for children between the ages of 5 and 6.

Procedure

The questionnaires for this study were administered between 2007 and 2008 by the principal investigator and four research assistants. The instrument used for this study were questionnaires adapted from the National Center for Chronic Disease Prevention and Health Promotion's *Healthy Youth* questionnaires for classroom research. The specific part of the questionnaires that were used were those that related to *classroom injuries prevention and safety questionnaires.* The open-ended questions that were used for the qualitative study were developed by the author. Participation was voluntary and consent forms were read by participants before the interviews and the completion of the questionnaires.

Coding

Two people were involved in the coding of the completed questionnaires. The coding involved an assessment of the content of the data (by the coders) with the intent of identifying common themes. All the themes identified were agreed upon by all the coders.

Data Analysis

For the quantitative analysis, association between binary categorical variables of interest was examined using chi-square test (df=1). The qualitative analysis was established from the answers to the open-ended questions from the interviews.

FINDINGS

The results of this study indicate that all research participants were female and aged between twenty-one and fifty-nine. Their mean age was 42.033 years and the standard deviation of their ages was 11.6 years with the median age of 42.50 years (see Table 1 for the age range of the participants).

Table 1. Participants' Age

Age Range	No of Participants
20- 30	19
31- 40	34
41- 50	25
51 -60	42

Furthermore, the results indicate that all surveyed participants taught injury prevention and safety lessons. The injury prevention and safety lessons taught were *fire safety*, *playground safety*, *water safety*, *emergency preparedness*, *sports protective equipment safety*, *pedestrian safety*, *motor vehicle occupant safety*, *poisoning safety*, *first aid*, and *gun safety*. Table 2 shows participants (in various age groups) and courses that they taught.

Table 2. Number of Participants Who Taught Specific Injury Lessons

Age Range	Number of Participants	Water-Safety		Emergency Preparedness		Pedestrian Safety		Motor Vehicle		Protective Equipment		First Aidm Safety		Poisoning Prevention		Gun Safety	
		Yes	No	Yes	No	Yes	No	Yes	No	Yes	No	Yes	No	Yes	No	Yes	No
20-30	19	13	6	13	6	10	9	9	10	13	6	4	15	3	16	2	17
31-40	34	15	19	24	10	29	5	30	4	22	12	7	27	8	26	5	29
41-50	25	10	15	12	13	14	11	18	7	14	11	6	19	7	18	5	20
51-60	42	7	35	16	26	37	5	33	9	16	26	13	29	12	30	3	39

Key: Yes = Did teach injuries lesson; No = Did not teach injuries lesson

Table 3. Health Background of Teachers Who Taught Injury Lessons

Age Range	HET	NHET	Water-Safety		Emergency Preparedness		Pedestrian Safety		Motor Vehicle		Protective Equipment		First Aidm Safety		Poisoning Prevention		Gun Safety	
			Yes	No	Yes	No	Yes	No	Yes	No	Yes	No	Yes	No	Yes	No	Yes	No
20-30	8	11	4	9	7	6	6	4	5	4	8	5	2	2	2	1	0	2
31-40	5	29	3	12	4	20	4	25	3	27	5	17	2	5	3	5	0	5
41-50	8	17	4	6	7	5	6	8	8	10	8	6	3	3	2	5	1	5
51-60	23	19	6	1	14	2	14	23	13	20	14	2	3	10	7	5	0	2

Key: Yes = Health background; No = No health background

With respect to the number of participants who taught specific injury prevention and safety topics, it was discovered that 100% of the surveyed participants taught *fire safety* and *playground safety*. Also, whereas 37.5% of respondents taught *water safety*, 62.5% did not ($\chi^2 = 7.5, p = .0006$).

Sixty-two percent of participants taught *emergency preparedness* and *sports protective equipment safety*, whereas 37.5% did not ($\chi^2 = 7.5$, $p = .0006$). Furthermore, whereas 75% of the population taught *pedestrian safety* as well as *motor vehicle occupant safety*, 25% did not ($\chi^2 = 30$, $p < .001$). Also, while 25% of the respondents taught *poisoning safety* and *first aid*, 75% did not ($\chi^2 = 30, p < .001$). Finally, only 12.5% of the respondents taught about *gun safety*, whereas 87.5% did not ($\chi^2 = 67.5, p <.001$).

Health Education Background

With regards to whether teachers who taught injury prevention lessons had training in health education, an observation of the data indicates that teachers without any health education background who were aged between 30 and 40 taught more injury prevention lessons than the teachers in the other age groups.

Also participants who indicated that they taught gun safety lessons were predominantly those who did not have any training in health education (see Table 3). From the data we observe that there was no difference in terms of number of years of experience and what teachers taught.

Water Safety

Of the 45 teachers who taught water safety, only 37.7% had health education training background; 53.3% did not. The age group that had a greater percentage of its population with a background in health education was the 51-60 group. About eighty-six percent (85.7%) of this group reported having a background in health education. Teachers who had the necessary health education background indicated that they were well prepared academically to teach water safety. For those without any training who taught water safety, the main reason given was fear of children drowning and hence the need to provide them with the basic training so as to minimize water-related accidents. Most of the teachers indicated that they knew how to swim and did not feel 'limited' or incompetent teaching about water safety. A teacher noted:

> I've been swimming all my life and therefore feel very confident teaching children about water safety, especially, the dangers that ponds and swimming pools pose to children. Taking water safety lessons from an expert could probably have increased my knowledge about water safety in general, but for my class, I think the personal experience I now have with water is enough.

A teacher who had training in water safety and who taught it to her class noted:

> I'm very confident in what I do because I took health lessons in which we talked about drowning and how to rescue people who are drowning, like a lifeguard, and stuff like that. These days most households in the suburbs have swimming pools so teaching about water safety is very important. Without proper academic and practical training it is impossible to teach about these safety issues in any proper way.

Emergency Preparedness

With teachers who taught emergency preparedness, there was no statistically significant difference between those with and those without an educational background in emergency preparedness (EP). Whereas 49.2% had prior educational training in EP, 50.8% did not. Some of the teachers with an educational background in emergency preparedness noted that they learned it through workshops. They indicated that the police, the fire department, and safety experts taught them about tornado drills, emergency evacuation, and things to do in terms of a threat to the lives of the school children. Teachers who taught EP noted that they taught it because of the danger and possibility of a terrorist threat or a disaster occurring and the need to ensure the children's safety. A teacher with an EP background noted:

> I teach my students about emergency safety all the time and we practice it with my students. In this day and age it will be naive to take emergency preparedness for granted. You never know when a terrorist action could take place so you have to stay on top of things.

A teacher with no formal background in EP who taught it to her students remarked:

> I'm yet to receive any practical training in emergency preparedness but I teach it anyway. It is such an important topic following the recent terrorist actions so you don't wait for training before you teach it. I teach them where (what room) to go to in case of fire or how to evacuate in case of an attack.

Pedestrian Safety

Three out of every four respondents taught pedestrian safety. Of the 90 who taught pedestrian safety, only 33% had any prior educational background in it; 67% did not have any training in it. All the respondents who indicated that they had prior training noted that they got their training through workshops and professional orientations. The main reason given by all the respondents (those with and those without prior training in pedestrian safety) for teaching pedestrian safety was to ensure that children respect other road users, avoid being run over by cars or bicycles, and know the importance of traffic lights and what each color (red, yellow, green, etc.) stands for. A teacher remarked:

> I teach these children about respect for other road users, about the need to walk or ride their bicycles on the correct side of the road, about the need to make sure an adult is present, and about the need to avoid risk and danger. You let them know the consequence of not following simple rules.

Motor Vehicle Safety

Motor vehicle safety, like pedestrian safety was taught by 75% of the respondents. Only 32.2% of the respondents who taught motor vehicle safety had any educational background in it. Like pedestrian safety, respondents who taught motor vehicle safety got their training in the subject through workshops. Furthermore, the respondents taught it to their kindergarten students because of the fear of possible vehicular accidents and the need for the children to be safe. They indicated that it was essential for the children to know about the importance of wearing seat belts and the appropriate way to wear them as well as the need to respect vehicular traffic and to know how to cross the road in the company of adults or a traffic crossing assistant. A participant noted:

> I make sure that they know safety tips on their finger tips so as to ensure their safety. I teach them about ways of crossing the road, the need to respect and obey the traffic signs and lights, and how to avoid being run over by bicycles and cars. Some of these young drivers drive at top speed even in neighborhoods and in the suburbs so it is important to help keep the children safe. Teaching motor vehicle safety is very important and every teacher must teach it.

Protective Equipment Safety

Out of the 65 teachers who taught protective equipment safety, 35 (53.8%) had prior educational background in it. Three said they learned about it in college, whereas the rest learned it at workshops. All the teachers who taught it taught about wearing helmets and knee protecting gear for riding bicycles. Two of the teachers taught of the use of mouth and nose masks by people with contagious diseases, masks for protecting oneself against certain allergens, and swimming gear to prevent drowning. A teacher noted that most accidents occur because children do not wear the appropriate protective equipment safety gear. She noted:

> Most accidents, whether bicycle related, auto related, or even in the swimming pools occur because parents and some of us, the teachers, do not make sure that the children are wearing the appropriate outfit. It is important to let the children know that protecting themselves with the appropriate equipment can save their lives. Every teacher must know about these and teach them to the children.

First Aid Safety

First aid safety was taught by only one in four (25%) of respondents. Two-thirds (67%) of those who taught first aid safety had no background in it. Of the 33% (n=10) who indicated they have an educational background in first aid safety, all learned it through workshops. All the 30 teachers who taught first aid safety indicated that they felt it was the most important safety tool to deal with injury. They also indicated that it was one area of safety that most of them did not feel competent and confident in teaching. The teachers indicated that they taught choking prevention, and treatment of nose bleeding and other forms of bleeding, among others. Some respondents called for workshops to assist them improve upon their knowledge in first aid safety in general and injury prevention in particular. A teacher noted:

> The scariest thing is when you see a child bleeding and you feel helpless. It is absolutely essential for every teacher to learn about first aid safety and to teach the children about basic first aid methods. You never know when a child could be a hero in helping to save the life of another child.

Poisoning Safety

Like first aid safety, only 25% of the respondents taught poisoning safety. Out of this figure, 46.7% had some educational background in it; 53.3% did not. What the teachers taught basically involved telling their parents or an adult or calling 911 if they or someone came into contact with poison. One teacher taught about poison ivy and another about lead poisoning. A common theme that ran across the teachers' responses was the need to make children aware of substances that had poison in them and the need to avoid such substances. A participant who did not teach about poisoning safety thought that teaching about such a topic will arouse the children's curiosity and subsequently cause some children to accidentally come into contact with it. She noted:

> I don't teach about poisoning safety although I have some background in it. Children are unpredictable so you have to be careful not to introduce certain topics since they may want to see if the danger you're talking about is real.

Gun Safety

Out of the 15 teachers who indicated that they taught about gun safety, only one had an educational background on firearms. When asked why they did not teach gun safety, some participants reported that it was lack of professional knowledge on gun safety that prevented them from teaching about guns. For such teachers, their preference was to invite professionals like policemen or military personnel as guest speakers to help children gain optimal knowledge about gun safety. Other participants also thought it was inappropriate to teach about guns at such an early age given children's high level of curiosity at that age and hence the danger of such children experimenting with guns if they are introduced to it. A teacher who did not teach gun safety wrote:

> I'm against teaching gun safety in schools because teaching it will definitely urge some children to look for guns and try using them. You know, children are curious and have the tendency to try out things and cause problems. I do not teach gun safety due to the issue of age appropriateness and elevating the fear factor. Also, I believe that in order to teach gun safety that it would have to be a co-operate decision not an individual one.

Teachers who taught gun safety believed that children should be aware of the dangers of guns. A participant wrote:

> I support teaching about gun safety in schools. What is happening these days is that kids, some as young as those in kindergarten, take guns to school and this is terrifying. There are shootings in many schools and you can never tell when it will happen in your backyard. It is therefore better to educate children about guns so that they understand the danger guns pose. It is important to educate children about guns so that they know what to do if they come across a gun.

Age Group

With regard to participants' age group and the kind of injury prevention topic(s) they taught, we observe from Table 2 that participants in age group 51-60 taught less water safety and gun safety although more teachers from that age group participated in the study than any other age group. We also observe that it was teachers in the 41-50 age group who did not teach emergency preparedness when compared with those in the other age groups. An observation of the data did not yield any reason(s) for the above-mentioned trend or course of action. Also, despite the fact that teachers between ages 31 and 40 were the second largest age group that participated in the study, the data showed that only two teachers from that age group taught the first aid safety lesson. We also learn from the data that only one teacher taught protective equipment safety from the 20-30 age group. Again, an observation of the data did not provide any reason to explain why respondents from above-mentioned age groups chose to teach certain topics and not others.

DISCUSSION AND CONCLUSION

The subject matter of this article has been to address injury prevention and safety lessons in kindergarten classrooms and to find out what teachers are doing about these important health issues.

In a study by the School Health Policies and Programs' arm of the Centers for Disease Control (2001) to assess school health policies and programs at the state, district, school, and classroom levels, the researchers noted that in spite of the need to prevent and deal with classroom injury, only 43% of elementary school teachers actually taught a topic or course on injury prevention. In this present study, from the utterances of participants we observed that some teachers' reason for not teaching injury prevention and safety issues in their kindergarten classrooms was their belief about the age-inappropriateness of some of the injury topics. Also, some teachers felt that the decision about whether or not a topic (such as gun safety) should be taught should be a cooperative effort between parents and educators. This study has also shown that lack of professional knowledge on the part of the teachers contributed to the teachers not teaching about some injury topics, especially gun safety. Teachers' inability to teach health education lessons due to lack of training is bolstered by other studies (see Ballard, White, & Glascoff, 1990).

From this study and others, we learn that it is important for kindergarten teachers to get appropriate training in order to help them impart important health knowledge on the children. This is particularly so given the fact that research has shown that proper training and ongoing support have the potential to equip teachers and prepare them to teach health topics efficiently (Hausman & Ruzek, 1995).

Also, since morbidity and mortality rates of injuries among children are high, the teaching of appropriate knowledge about injuries and safety from the children's schools may curtail such incidents now and in the future. This is particularly true given the fact that research has indicated that the experiences that children gain at schools are important in establishing their health behaviors in their later years (Nutbeam, Smith, Moore, & Bauman, 1993).

Furthermore, given the fact that participants in this research taught injury lessons on the average for less than an hour a week, it is essential for teachers to note that regular instructions on health education in general and on injury and safety in particular, based on all three learning domains (cognitive, affective, psychomotor) and taught at least fifty hours per year, is needed before any considerable changes could be made in children's attitudes and behaviors (English & Sancho, 1990). It is particularly recommended that teachers take note of the required number of hours needed for appropriate health instruction.

In sum, kindergarten teachers should spend more time in teaching children about injury prevention in order to prepare them for their adolescent years and to possibly reduce the morbidity and mortality rates among children.

SIGNIFICANCE

This study enlightens kindergarten teachers on injury prevention and safety topics that other colleagues have been focusing on and what needs to be done to improve children's knowledge and skills on injury prevention and safety issues. Health skills and knowledge are important in improving children's health behavior (Nutbeam *et al.*, 1993) and this research adds to that body of knowledge.

REFERENCES

Ballard, D., White, D., & Glascoff, M. (1990). AIDS/HIV education for pre-service elementary school teachers. *Journal of School Health*, 60, 262-265.

Center for Disease Control and Prevention's School Health Policies and Programs Study (2001). Accident and unintentional injury prevention. *Journal of School Health, 71*(7).

Dal Santo, J. A., Goodman, R. M., Glik, D., & Jackson, K. (2004). Childhood unintentional injuries: Factors predicting injury risk among preschoolers. *Journal of Pediatric Psychology, 29*(4), 273-283.

Dye, J. F., Schatz, I. M., Rosenberg, B. A., & Coleman, S. T. (2000). Constant comparison method: A kaleidoscope of data. *The Qualitative Report, 4*(1/2).

English, J., & Sancho, A. (1990). *Criteria for comprehensive health education curricula.* Los Alamitos, CA: Comprehensive Health Education Program, Southwest Regional Laboratory.

Hausman, A. J., & Ruzek, S. B. (1995). Implementation of comprehensive school health education in elementary schools: Focus on teacher concerns. *Journal of School Health. 65*(3), 81-86.

Kendrick, D., Coupland, C., Mulvaney, C., Simpson, J., Smith, S. J., Sutton, A., Watson, M., & Woods, A. (2007). Home safety education and provision of safety equipment for injury prevention. *Cochrane Database of Systematic Reviews, 1*, CD005014.

Kim, M. H., Subramanian, S. V., Kawachi, I., & Kim, C. Y. (2007). Association between childhood fatal injuries and socioeconomic position at individual and area levels: A multilevel study. *Journal of Epidemiology and Community Health, 61*, 135-140.

Knoff, H. M. (2001). *The Stop and Think Social Skills Program.* Boston, MA: Sopris West.

Nutbeam, D., Smith, C., Moore, L, & Bauman, A. (1993). Warning! Schools can damage your health: Alienation from school and its impact on health behaviour. *Journal of Paediatrics and Child Health, 29*(1), 25-30.

Pickett, W., Ardern, C., & Brison, R. J. (2001). A population-based study of potential brain injuries requiring emergency care. *Canadian Medical Association Journal, 165*(3), 288-292.

Schwebel, D. C., Brezausek, C. M., & Belsky, J. (2006). Does time spent in child care influence risk for unintentional injury? *Journal of Pediatric Psychology*, 31(2), 184-193.

Spinks, A. B., McClure, R. J., Bain, C., & Macpherson, A. K. 2006. Quantifying the association between physical activity and injury in primary school-aged children. *Pediatrics, 118*(1), E45-E50.

Strauss, A., & Corbin, J. (1998). *Basics of qualitative research: Techniques and procedures for developing grounded theory* (2nd ed.). Thousand Oaks, CA: Sage.

Chapter 4

HEALTH ACTIVITIES IN PRESCHOOL CLASSROOMS: DO PRESCHOOL CHILDREN GET ENOUGH INFORMATION ABOUT HEALTHY LIVING BEHAVIOR IN THEIR CLASSROOMS?

ABSTRACT

The purpose of this chapter was to analyze qualitatively what health-related activities that 42 preschool teachers in some Indiana preschools incorporated in their classroom. Pre-school teachers were asked to complete a questionnaire requesting them to indicate what health-related activities they were incorporating into their classroom routines and whether such activities were enough to help the children receive sufficient information about healthy living behavior. The study discovered that the most taught health-related activities were hand washing, discussion on germs, "my pyramid", food safety, yoga, outside play, and keeping harmful things out of the mouth. The least taught health-related activities were proper use of the bathroom, exercise videos, and spitting. Although teachers generally viewed the incorporation of health-related activities into their class schedules as very important, it was discovered that not every teacher reported incorporating health-related activities in their classrooms. The study recommends that all important stakeholders in preschool education come together in order to come up with strategies that will ensure adequate training in Health Education for preschool teachers to guarantee integration of appropriate health-related materials in the preschool classroom.

INTRODUCTION

Childhood health problems especially obesity and chronic overweight (Hedley et al., 2004; Ogden, Carrol & Flegal, 2003) have become endemic in children due to a decline in physical activity (Young, et al., 2007).

With respect to the connection between nutrition and physical health, scholarship on nutrition indicates that improper nutrition weakens the body's immune system (Suttajit, 2007) thereby making the body prone to disease (Duerksen et al., 2007). The above situation can be problematic given the fact that children who are obese and inactive often grow up to become obese (Patrick & Nicklas, 2005) and inactive adults (Melville et al., 2007) and can go on to develop dangerous diseases like hypertension, diabetes, and even cancer (Magarey et. al., 2003).

On personal cleanliness, studies show that lack of proper cleanliness (such as dirty or cluttered housing, tooth decay, improper washing of hands, among others), leads to the spread of disease and allergens (Peters et al. 2007). Given the above studies, it is surprising to observe the dearth of scholarship on actual health-related activities that preschool teachers incorporate into their daily classroom activities. The situation is even more surprising given the importance educators attach to preschool and childcare centers in the promotion of child health.

A study of the physical activity patterns and associated variables of Anglo-American and Mexican-American 4-year-old children from low to middle socioeconomic families showed ethnic differences for both physical activity and environmental variables (McKenzie et al. (1992). The researchers discovered that habitual physical activity in children is related to physical fitness and appears to mediate cardiovascular disease risk factors. The authors found significant correlations between children's activity patterns at home and during recess at school. Specifically, they found out that Mexican-American preschool children were less active than Anglo-American preschool children at home and during recess at school. Their findings give further credence to the notion that physical activity lifestyle habits may be established in early childhood cognizant of the fact that young children rapidly gain health and safety knowledge if such knowledge is communicated to them during early years. This makes preschool an important time for caregivers to incorporate health-promoting behaviors into children's lifestyles.

Other studies on preschool health have focused on perceptions of health status and play activities in parents of overweight toddlers and preschoolers (Rich et al., 2005). A study of Hispanic toddlers and preschoolers from lower socioeconomic background, for example, showed an increase in childhood overweight among the participants surveyed in their study. To their surprise, the authors discovered that most participants believed their child was healthy and half were unconcerned about their child's weight. The researchers learned that access to an outside play area was related to amount of active play activities. They concluded by calling on health professionals to partner with parents in order to address childhood obesity.

In a study that examined, among other things, the developmental appropriateness and cultural sensitivity of school-based prevention programs aimed specifically at symptom reduction or behavior promotion, the authors (Humphries & Keenan, 2006) expressed surprise at the relatively few school-based prevention programs targeted for preschoolers despite the fact that prevention, if started in early years, tends to reach maximum effectiveness. Despite the fact that many health problems are considered alterable if intervention is started in childhood (Mobley, 1996), and given the important role the preschool setting plays in children's health, little is known about health knowledge in preschool settings in general, and health-related activities in preschool classrooms in particular.

Purpose

Given the importance educators attach to preschool and childcare centers in the promotion of child health and in view of the dearth of scholarly work health related activities done in preschool classrooms, the purpose of this study is to fill that knowledge gap by attempting to answer the following research questions:

What kind of activities (health-related) do preschool teachers incorporate in their classrooms and whether such Information is enough about healthy living?

Based on the principle findings, recommendations will be made to educators in order to help provide preschool children with the appropriate health knowledge and skills that will subsequently lead to the improvement of preschool children's health and overall wellbeing.

METHODOLOGY

Procedure

Indiana Preschool teachers were recruited upon approval from Indiana University's Institutional Review Board. The teachers who expressed interest in participating in the research and who were Lead Teachers or Assistant Teachers were given questionnaires to complete. Schools from which the surveyed participants were recruited were selected by convenience and were mainly within a fifty-mile radius from Indianapolis. The study instrument requested participants to indicate what health-related topics or activities they incorporated into their classroom schedules, and why they included them in their class schedules. In order to ascertain the reliability of what was indicated on the questionnaires, participants were asked to complete the questionnaires that focused on the open-ended questions again a month later. The questionnaires were administered between May 2006 and January 2007. Participation was voluntary.

RESULTS

Two hundred and five questionnaires were sent out and 112 were completed. Out of the 112 returned surveys, forty-two were selected for this qualitative study because besides completing the closed-ended questionnaires, the respondents completely and appropriately answered the open-ended questions that required them to provide reasons for incorporating health-related topics in their classrooms. Information from the closed-ended questions in all the 112 returned surveys is discussed in Obeng (2008).

The findings are grouped under three broad health-related activities: (a) Personal hygiene, (b) Food, and (c) Exercise.

Table 1. Major Health Activities

Major Health Topics/ Activities	# Of Respondents	%
Personal hygiene	42	100
Food	37	88.1
Exercise	30	71.4

FINDINGS AND DISCUSSION

Personal Hygiene

All 42 respondents (100%) reported personal cleanliness as a health-related activity performed in their classrooms. The least-incorporated health activities in the classrooms were proper use of the bathroom and keeping harmful things out of the mouth. With respect to activities involving keeping harmful things out of the mouth, the teachers indicated that they talked about things that children should not put into their mouth and nose. The most mentioned activity teachers incorporated into their class was hand washing. Fourteen of the surveyed participants incorporated hand washing into their class activities.

A participant indicated that:

> Hand washing is a good activity that every teacher needs to encourage in their classrooms. Children need to wash their hand several times to avert germs.

Food

Although a majority of the preschool teachers incorporated activities on food in their classroom schedules, some of them did not do it on a daily basis.

A participant noted that:

> We barely get any time to introduce how to choose healthy food in our daily classroom activities because there are so many things to do within the hours that the children are with us.

Exercise

At least a majority of teachers in the sample reported doing exercise-related activities. The teacher's indicated that they did various exercise activities with children.

One teacher wrote:

> Exercise is good for children. It helps them make friends and cooperate with others children. Exercise is a cooperative activity that helps them socialized with their schoolmates.

A close attention to the excerpts cited in the previous sections and to the results of the survey demonstrates that most of the teachers are generally aware of the benefits of incorporating health-related activities into their daily classroom routines and therefore place a high premium on some of the activities. Specifically, reasons given by the preschool teachers for incorporating the health-related activities in their class schedules point to their awareness of the health benefits of such activities and the consequences of not incorporating them in their lessons.

The survey findings demonstrate that despite the fact that the teachers are generally aware of specific health activities and their benefits to the children, not all teachers integrated such health-related activities in their normal class schedules and some teachers who integrated them did so sparingly. Thus, there was no uniformity and consistency in type of activities incorporated and how often such activities were incorporated in the teachers' schedules. For example, although all 42 participants viewed the incorporation of health-related activities into class schedules as very important, not all viewed activities on food and exercise as equally important. On personal hygiene, for example, not all teachers did activities on personal hygiene. This has implications for practice. Specifically, it points to the need for pre-school teachers' attention to be drawn to the fact that all health activities are important. Furthermore, given the prevalence of obesity and Type 2 diabetes in children, and despite the preponderance of scholarship demonstrating the fact that good health and nutrition provide the biological basis for adequate physical activity that may improve cognitive development, social interactions, economic productivity, and the quality of life of an individual or a population (Torun B, 1989) only few of the teachers who did activities on nutrition actually incorporated activities on a daily basis. Whereas all the surveyed participants paid attention to personal cleanliness not all did activities relating to exercise. These lapses have implications for teacher-educators. Specifically, it calls on teacher-educators to closely examine the connection between children's health status and access to good nutrition and actual play activities and to subsequently emphasize this in the teacher-training curriculum. For preschool teachers, this calls for the incorporation of more activities on different facets of nutrition and different types of exercise into their daily class routines.

Moreover, the fact that some teachers paid little or no attention to some activities, points to the fact that it is important for colleges and universities to assist all teachers to gain adequate training in health education. It is also important that all preschool directors come together to come up with strategies that will ensure adequate children-educators ratio in order to guarantee appropriate and competent supervision of the children in childcare.

LIMITATION OF STUDY

The survey relied entirely on teachers' self-reports via questionnaires and through interviews. No visits were made to the schools to verify whether the teachers actually incorporated any of the self-reported activities. Also, although the anonymity of the survey would act against over- or under-reporting on the part of teachers, one cannot rule out such over- or under-reporting. Finally, a limitation to the method for selecting participants is the possibility of self-selection bias.

CONCLUSION

From the data and the above discussion, it could be concluded that the preschool teachers surveyed for this study recognize the fact that an incorporation of health-related activities into their class schedules performs an important role in preschoolers' health. Specifically, the teachers recognize the fact that doing health-related activities generally helps to keep the children fit and consequently assist society in avoiding the spread of diseases, and preventable possible deaths.

Also by helping to instill personal cleanliness, the teachers have by their actions shown the great role they play in helping to keep preschoolers safe and sound. There is no doubt that early years constitute the best time for teaching children about good eating habits and broad social and cognitive skills that are necessary for healthy and decent living and this study has shown the role teachers can play toward the accomplishment of the above goals.

Finally, to ensure that preschool teachers effectively perform their role of instilling living a healthy lifestyle in the children they teach, it is incumbent on colleges and universities, and the entire society to assist them by making the necessary tools and training available to them; by so doing we can avert some problems in the health of children.

Implications for Practice

Teachers need to be informed through workshops about health education training. Even if some teachers choose not to take advantage of such workshops, it is important for teacher-trainers to make them available and accessible to all teachers. In addition to this, the school districts need to mount an educational campaign to communicate with teachers about the health-related education training It may also be important for teachers to invite experts like nurses, fire marshals, yoga experts, and nutritionists to their classrooms to help intensify health education at this early level of education cognizant of the fact that it is at such a stage that children begin to actually learn to build a lifestyle that will either help or hurt them in the future.

References

Duerksen, S. C., Elder, J. P., Arredondo, E. M., Ayala, G. X., Slymen, D. J., Campbell, N. R., & Baquero, B. (2007). Family restaurant choices are associated with child and adult overweight status in Mexican-American families. *Journal of the American Dietetic Association, 107*(5), 849-853.

Hedley, A. A., Ogden, C. L., Johnson, C. LCarroll,M.D; Curtin,L. Flegal, K.MR. (2004). Prevalence of overweight and obesity among US children, adolescents, and adults, 1999-2002. *JAMA*, 291(23), 2847-2850.

Humphries, M. L. & Keenan, K. E. (2006). Theoretical, developmental and cultural orientations of school-based prevention programs for preschoolers. *Clinical Child and Family Psychology Review* 9(2), 135-148.

Magarey, A. M., Daniels, L. A., Boulton, T. J., Cockington, R. A. (2003). Predicting obesity in early adulthood from childhood and parental obesity. *International Journal of Obesity and Related Metabolism Disorders, 27,* 505-513.

McKenzie, T. L., Sallis, J. F., Nader, P. R., Broyles, S. L., & Nelson, J. A. (1992). Anglo-American and Mexican-American preschoolers at home and at recess - activity patterns and environmental-influences. *Journal of Developmental and Behavioral Pediatrics 13*(3), 173-180.

Melville, C. A., Hamilton, S., Hankey, C. R., Miller, S., & Boyle, S. (2007). The prevalence and determinants of obesity in adults with intellectual disabilities. *Obesity Reviews 8*(3), 223-230.

Mobley, C. E. (1996). Assessment of health knowledge in preschoolers. *Children's Health Care 25*(1), 11-18

Ogden, C. L., Carroll, M. D., Flegal, K. M. (2003). Epidemiologic trends in overweight and obesity. *Endocrinol Metab Clin North Am*erica *32*, 741-760.

Patrick, H., Nicklas, T. A. (2005). A review of Family and social determinants of children's eating patterns and diet quality. *Journal of the American College of Nutrition, 24*(2), 83-92.

Peters, J. L., Levi, J. I., Rogers, C. A., Burge, H. A., & Spengler, J. D. (2007). Determinants of allergen concentrations in apartments of asthmatic children living in public housing. *Journal of Urban Health-Bulletin of the New York Academy of Medicine, 84* (2), 185-197.

Rich, S. S., DiMarco, N. M., Essery, E. V., Anderson, E., & Sanborn, C. F. (2005). Perceptions of health status and play activities in parents of overweight Hispanic toddlers and preschoolers. *Family & Community Health 28*(2), 130-141.

Stolley, M. R., Fitzgibon, M.L., Dyer, A., Horn, L. V., Kaufer-Christoffel, K., & Schiffer, L. (2003). Hip-Hop to Health Jr., an obesity prevention program for minority preschool children: Baseline characteristics of participants. *Preventive Medicine, 36*, 320-329.

Suttajit, M. (2007). Advances in nutrition support for quality of life in HIV+/AIDS. *Asia Pacific Journal of Clinical Nutrition, 16,* 318-322.

Torun, B. (1989). Increase of physical-activity by improvement of nutritional-status. *Archivos Latinoamericanos De Nutricion, 39*(3), 308-326.

Young, D. R., Felton, G. M., Elder, J. P., Johnson, C; Lee, J; Kubik, M. (2007). Policies and opportunities for physical activity in middle school environments. *Journal of School Health, 77*(1), 41-47.

Chapter 5

FAMILIES WITH CHILDREN WITH SPECIAL NEEDS

ABSTRACT

The aim of this chapter is to elicit parents' reports about the stresses associated with caring for children with disabilities. There were 15 mothers with children with disabilities in the study. The results suggest that no matter the level of a child's health problem the whole family's life is adversely affected. Participants' utterances also suggest that despite the great deal of burden placed on the parents by their children's health problems the parents did not get much help from outside and that worsened their burden.

INTRODUCTION

Lack of knowledge and proper understanding about diseases that lead to chronic health problems as well as ways that such diseases manifest themselves in individuals have contributed to people faced by such problems being stigmatized (Obeng, C 2007). Silk et al. (2000) attest to the fact that children with health problems, especially those with mental illness, have only recently begun to be studied as separate from adults.

Society's negative attitude toward children with health problems, especially those with mental health problems, has tremendous influence on the children and their families. The above claim is bolstered by Kinsella and Anderson's (1996) study in which they note that, due to the interdependence that exists within family systems, there is the tendency for each member of a family to be affected by a child's health problem. This suggests that it is important to look at the entire family, not only the child who is sick.

This chapter, therefore, examines the specific experiences that some families (mothers) of chronically ill children go through and how, through their stories, we can explore coping strategies they consider workable and/or appropriate to their unique circumstances.

PROCEDURE

This study used the *narrative methodology* approach (variously referred to as *narrative inquiry)* (see Patton, 1990; and Connelly & Clandinin, 1990). The use of the *Narrative inquiry* approach was appropriate for this work because it allowed the data to be closely examined into various analytical categories; comparisons were made for similarities and differences. Detailed analyses of participants' utterances were made in order to find out the mothers' perspectives in caring for their children with chronic health problems.

The data were collected between 2004 and 2007. Twenty parents were contacted, and fifteen women accepted the invitation to participate in the study. Participants were from the Midwest in the United States.

The instrument was designed to solicit information related to parents' experiences in caring for their children as well as coping strategies that they used in their homes to help their children with disabilities.

All interviews were conducted by the author and a colleague. In total, fifteen parents participated in the research. Two people, paying attention to such issues as the nature of the disabilities and coping strategies of the families, coded the data. The analysis done in this study involves verbatim quotations from participants as well as thematic interpretation

RESULTS

Participants and their children information are in Table 1 below.

Table 1. Summary of reported health problems

Parents	Number of health problems diagnosed	Age when disability was diagnosed by a professional	Identified health problem
A	4	8	Seizure disorder, cerebral palsy, heart disease
B	1	1.5	Autism
C	3	13	Obsessive compulsive disorder, personality disorder, anxiety disorder
D	1	At birth	Cerebral palsy, vertebral anomalies, history of heart murmur, profound to severe hearing loss in both ears, a seizure disorder, paralyzed right side of face, malformed right ear, malformed jaw, small size (in 3rd percentile for height/weight), low muscle tone, loose joints, hypernasality in speech, and growth hormone deficiency
E	3	6	Learning disability in written language, speech delay, ADHD
F	3	11	food allergies
G	3	At birth	Congenital heart disease, language delay, seizures
H	2	At birth	Down's syndrome
I	2	5.5 month	Physical problems, lissencephaly
J	6	9	Epilepsy
K	4	5	Mental retardation, epilepsy
L	3	At birth	Fetal alcohol syndrome
N	4	4	Asthma
M	2	7	Diabetes
O	4	3	Obsessive compulsive disorder, allergies

An observation of the data confirms that it was health professionals who identified most research participants' children's health problems. Parents whose children were diagnosed with multiple health problems complained of poor quality of life in the form of unending problems and uncertainty. For example, a parent whose child was diagnosed with multiple health problems at birth noted:

> The first week her face looks abnormal. The second week it was breathing problems. After her first birthday we saw that she had a serious balance problem and she also had a seizure after one year ten months. In addition she had language delay; we were having difficulty with toilet training also. Her problems keep on adding and we are [sic] not sure the exact number of problems that she had.

Another respondent said:

> Every little noise will wake her up including probably the noise that comes from the fall of a tooth stick. You will put her to bed thinking that you will have some time for rest but by the time you get to your bedroom she is already up.

Another observation made from the transcripts was that although people generally sympathized with families with children suffering from chronic health problems, there was not much real support for them (the families) in the areas of a Case Manager, babysitting, and health insurance. The lack of appropriate support placed a considerable burden on the families and also affected their quality of life. For example, a participant reported that her child's abnormality had gravely affected her emotional health. Almost in tears, she remarked:

> People seem to sympathize with you when they know that you have a child with disabilities. They often use words that seem they will give you all the help you will need in this world when having conversation with them. But when they hear the word heart disease, cerebral parsley [sic]; all potential helpers are not willing to take care of your child, they then find unreasonable excuses to support why they will not be able to help. This situation is very frustrating because people dwell so much on the child disabilities not the good things that they will be able to do.

Another participant said:

> No support groups for families with children with special needs . . . or when one is started, it lasts for a very short period of time.

Some participants reported that their quality of life was being adversely impacted by their children's illness. They noted that they were weighed down by the amount of time they spent on such events as doctor visits, therapies, surgeries, tests, follow-up conversations, scheduling phone calls, and travel to and from such activities that related to medical care for their children.

Some parents suggested that having a director of child's health care (a Case Manager) with the responsibility of assisting families or acting as a liaison between families and the various healthcare units would help reduce the amount of providers that they had to deal with. The respondents noted that such a director could oversee the care and subsequently help make clinical appointments, do the necessary paperwork, file insurance claims, communicate with the parents, and follow the progress of the child. Furthermore, such a director, the respondents contended, could let the families know about resources available to them and even help set up things like family therapy, respite care, and special educational opportunities that are so essential to managing and/or coping with the children's healthcare needs.

As one of the participant reported:

> Our daughter is being followed by thirteen doctors and two additional therapists. Handling the scheduling and paperwork for all of those is challenging. It is not uncommon for paperwork issues to take hours on the phone to resolve.

Participants also reported not receiving help in babysitting their children, a situation that impacted their lives negatively since it caused them to be fatigued and depressed. Specifically, we learned from the participants' narratives that there was a great need for help in terms of babysitting in order to give them a break. The mothers indicated that they were frustrated because they did not receive the help they so desperately needed.

Another factor that caused the quality of life of the families to be poor was low family income and hence their inability to secure appropriate health insurance. Participants' narratives revealed a common trend in which parents were unable to find a suitable insurance plan even after their child's health problem(s) was/were diagnosed. As one parent put it:

> We've always been in debt ever since our daughter's disease was diagnosed. It's that simple it is impossible to find a perfect insurance to cover one's debts.

The surveyed parents who had no health insurance noted that the absence of health insurance added to their stressed lives since they spent hours thinking about what to do should their child's condition worsened. The rather difficult situation in which the parents found themselves made planning ordinary routinized activities as well as financial planning a nightmare.

Also, some of the parents noted that their children's health problems were many and/or occurred in succession, making it impossible for them to determine what the nature of one problem was or the next problem would be and from where they could possibly get help. Such uncertainty made it impossible to do any meaningful planning and hence negatively impacted their quality of life.

A majority of the mothers alluded, in their narratives, to the fact that because they spent so much time with their children, and also because of the nature of their children's problems, any long-term relationship was practically impossible. A participant reported that her divorce was caused by her husband and also by the fact that she and the husband could not have time for each other because of the child's special health condition. She noted:

> There is always no time to spend with anybody; you are always finding ways of solving your child's problems. Any man who seems to be interested in long relationship quits after few years because of constant problems in the home.

Two parents also reported the following about their marriages breaking down because of their children's chronic health problems. One said:

> At least 2 of my divorces have something to do with the strife caused either directly or indirectly by this child. The stress on the family is enormous and chronic. There's no escape.

The other parent noted:

> The stress of caring for her significantly reduced the quality of our marital relationship. We separated permanently when our daughter was six years old.

Some parents complained of financial burdens, being stigmatized by neighbors and other people, not knowing what to do, sibling non-coherence, and being stressed out due to a combination of social and emotional factors.

A parent observed:

> It is emotionally challenging to watch our daughter suffer physically and socially. She has had numerous hospitalizations and surgeries and has suffered considerably since birth. Her care has been challenging for us. The stress has impacted our wider social lives (we lost contact with most of our friends during our child's first three years). Her care has been mostly covered by insurance, but non-covered expenses have provided significant financial burdens to us. Our daughter is now in first grade and yet to experience much expected social stigmatization from her physical and social differences. Around this, we have significant anticipatory stress.

Another participant also said:

> The unpredictability of his episodes of anger, meanness and aggressiveness. His seeming lack of empathy for others. Also, his siblings have almost no relationship with their brother because he seems uninterested or unable to attach to them.

Participants indicated that despite the fact that their children were sometimes mean to them and to their siblings, they (the participants) avoided vengeance; rather, they looked for ways to avoid issues and events that triggered the children's unusual behavior. Participants also made every effort to protect their other children so that their health problems did not affect the quality of life that they led.

Another factor that positively impacted the quality of life of the families was the availability of books and Internet resources that helped them in coping with their unique situations. Some of the parents made constant attempts to look for information concerning their children's illness from books and information on the worldwide web. According to such parents, the above-mentioned resources gave them bits and pieces of information or ideas about what to look for in the child's health problems. Some of the parents reported that they were guided by such literature on what actions to take during a critical episode. Such knowledge helped to prepare them emotionally for unexpected erratic behavior on the part of their children.

Other parents noted that information from professionals, and sometimes from parents with older children with similar health problems as their child, helped them to cope with their children's health problems. Parents gave such short comments as:

> "Get support and get it early."
> "Become an expert in your child's disability."
> "Learn how to be an advocate for your child, in every way."
> "Surround yourself with people who support you and your child."
> "Just be as supportive and open to new ideas."

Finally, we learned from the transcripts that some of the children with health problems had important skill(s) that even normal children did not have. However, the parents noted that because of society's misunderstanding of their children's illness, such skills and talents were totally ignored; a situation that the parents said negatively affected their quality of life because it led them to being stressed more.

DISCUSSION

On the nature and extent of health problems, the responses cited in the previous section and other similar responses found in the data show the discomfort that the children and their parents went through. It could be inferred from the responses that the children's illnesses had a considerable negative impact on the quality of life of the children and that of their parents. Specifically, through the parents' narratives they complained of desperation, emotional and mental problems, sleeplessness, and plain suffering—problems also identified in Berntsson and Gustafsson's (2000) study of psychosomatic issues associated with Swedish school children with chronic illness and their illness' impact of their families.

An important observation from the results had to do with the low quality of life of the families brought about by the not-so-strong family economy. The weak financial standing of some of the parents was brought about by their inability to work full-time because they had to spend long hours with their children. Also, they received insufficient and/or inappropriate support in the areas of Case Management, babysitting, and health insurance. The results showed further that the above situation placed considerable socio-emotional and cognitive burdens on the families leading to frustration and a sense of helplessness and hopelessness. The above finding is not unique to the population studied in this research.

Berntsson and Gustafsson's (2000) study also showed how children's illness impacted their mothers' health and their families' finances, leading them to rightfully call for viewing and dealing with children's mental or emotional health within the context of the child, the family, and the society.

In the present study, it is suggested that providing appropriate and/or adequate assistance to the families such as providing them with a case worker who will let them know about resources available to them and even help set up things like family therapy, respite care, and special educational opportunities that are so essential to managing and/or coping with the children's healthcare will ease the stress and burden on them thereby improving their quality of life.

With respect to the parents' inability to find suitable health insurance after their child had been diagnosed with a chronic illness, we glean from the results that such a situation throws the families into perpetual debt and subsequently makes them suffer from undue and excessive stress. Their stressful lives by and large render them incapable of planning their lives meaningfully and hence seeing the quality of their lives significantly decrease.

Another aspect of quality of life suffered by the surveyed parents had to do with the impact of their stressed lives on their marriages. The fact that a majority the women surveyed in the study were divorced and in view of the fact that some of them blamed their divorce on their children's illness and the stress associated with caring for such children has implications for how the mental health of families dealing with children who have chronic illnesses should be viewed and/or handled. In particular, it calls on society to critically examine the root cause of family stress and how necessary and important it is to employ a family-centered mental health management Berntsson and Gustafsson (2000); Kinsella and Anderson (1996).

Other problems that negatively impacted the quality of life of the families were their stigmatization by neighbors and other members of the society and poor sense of coherence. From the results (participants' excerpts) we learned that the stigmatization and poor sense of coherence led to excessive stress and other socio-emotional problems, a situation also identified by Groholt et al. (2003) in their study in some Nordic countries. In this present study, the fact that the parents looked for ways to avoid issues and events that triggered the children's unusual behavior and also made every effort to protect their other children so that their sick children's health problems did not affect the quality of life that they led, points to the high level of endurance and/or resilience of the families and their desire to lead 'normal' lives despite their difficult circumstances. It also points to how essential it is to make the parents in particular, and the entire family in general, part of the overall management of children's health. Specifically, as primary caregivers, the family plays a significant role, not only in assisting with the diagnosing of their child's health problems, but also by being the first responders to any critical health episode or event and by being the primary institution in the healthcare delivery.

Given the help the families received from books and Internet resources toward improving their quality of life, it could be argued that it is high time social workers, healthcare delivery organizations, and the government paid attention to the nature and extent of materials made available online and in libraries for families dealing with children who have health problems. Making the right and relevant literature available in audio, video/visual, and textual form on the worldwide web and making such websites known to families will go a long way to ease the burden of families.

From the above discussion, we learn that for parents with children with health problems no help is considered too little. It is however important to note that a lot more education about children's health problems is necessary not only for the surveyed parents but for every parent. More importantly, parents need to be properly informed about what is on the web and the danger that some information could pose to the effective management of their children's health problems.

Finally, based on the results in the previous section, it is important to end this section on cautious note. In particular, the fact that some of the children with health problems had important skill(s) that most so-called mainstream or 'normal' children did not have, but because of society's misunderstanding of their illness, such skills and talents were totally ignored, suggests that if society gives them an equal chance as is given to other children, there could be an improvement in the quality of life of these children and their families. Ignoring the children's skills and dwelling on the negative aspects of the health problems will do nothing but add to the affected families' woes and decrease their quality of life.

SUMMARY AND RECOMMENDATIONS

This study has shown that the health problems of chronically ill children have the potential to impact their parents' personal, social, and marriage lives. Two positive discoveries made in this study were parents' unconditional love for their children and the life and academic skills of some of the children. Specifically, this study showed that most of the surveyed parents were patient, tolerant, and loving toward their children no matter the situation in which they found themselves. The parents' willingness to sacrifice their peace, comfort, and even social and matrimonial necessities for the welfare of their children suggest that if appropriate help is given, the lives of the children and those of their parents will be improved considerably.

This study recommends that people should look at the positive side of the lives of such children and offer the parents and the children the necessary help they need in order to be able to manage their daily routines.

Finally, this study recommends the need to learn more about children's health problems in order to do away with stereotypes and stigmatizations attached to them. It is also recommended that society in general, and social workers in particular, offer the necessary help needed by parents with children who have health problems in order to help them cope with the challenges they face daily. Specifically, having case managers to assist parents, providing the right coping resources, and creating an appropriate and/or enabling learning atmosphere for the children will lessen the mothers' burden and improve the children's lives.

REFERENCES

Berntsson, L. T. & Gustafsson, J. E. (2000). Determinants of psychosomatic complaints in Swedish schoolchildren aged seven to twelve years. *Scandinavian Journal Public Health*, *28*(4), 283-93.

Connelly, F. M. & Clandinin DJ. (1990). Stories of experience and narrative inquiry. *Educational Researcher 19*(5), 2-14.

Groholt, E. K., Stigum, H., Nordhagen, R., & Kohler, L. (2003). Is parental sense of coherence associated with child health? *European Journal Public Health, 13*(3), 195-201.

Kinsella, K. & Anderson, R. (1996). Coping skills, strengths, and needs as perceived by adult offspring and siblings of people with mental illness: a retrospective study. *Psychiatry Rehabilitation Journal, 20,* 24-32.

Obeng, C. S. (2007). Perceptions of epilepsy in a family. In *HIV/AIDS, illness and African well-being* (Toyin, F., Heaton, M. ed.), Rochester University Press, Rochester, 57-71.

Silk J, Nath S, Siegel L, Kendall P. Conceptualizing mental disorders in children: where have we been and where are we going? *Developmental Psychopathology* 2000; 12: 713-35.

Turnbull, A. P., Brown, I., Turnbull, H. R. eds. (2001). *Family quality of life: an international perspective*, American Association on Mental Retardation, Washington, DC.

Chapter 6

INCLUSION OF CHILDREN WITH DISABILITIES IN THE CLASSROOM

ABSTRACT

This chapter presents a brief but lucid review of the literature on inclusion paying particular attention to what it is and why people are striving toward it. This is followed by a review of the relevant information on inclusion in the Ghanaian educational system. The final section is a brief conclusion.

LITERATURE REVIEW ON INCLUSION IN THE UNITED STATES

Sailor (1991: 10) defines inclusion as 'making all students attend schools to which they would go if they had no disability, recognizing the fact that a natural proportion of students with learning disabilities occur at each school site, implementing a zero rejection philosophy to ensure that no student would be excluded based on type or extent of disability, ensuring that school and general education placements are age and grade appropriate without there being no self-contained special education classes operative at the school site, ensuring that cooperative learning and peer instructional methods receive significant use in general instructional practice at the school site, and ensuring that special education supports are provided within the context of the GEC and in other integrated environment'. According to Morgan (1991:2), full inclusion means that all children must be educated in supported, heterogeneous, age-appropriate, natural, child-focused classrooms, schools and community environments for the purpose of preparing them for full participation in a diverse and integrated society. Morgan (ibid:10) notes that a full inclusive program must have the following characteristics: (a) all students attend schools to which they would go if they had no disability; (b) a natural proportion of students with disabilities occurs at each school site; (c) a zero rejection philosophy exists so that typically no student would be excluded on the basis of type or extent of disability; (d) school and general education placements are age- gender-appropriate, with no self-contained special education classes operative at the school site; (e) cooperative learning and peer instructional methods receive significant use in general instructional practice at the school site; and (f) special education supports are provided within the context of general education class and in other integrated environment. From the above scholarly definitions, inclusion involves educating all students in the same regular classrooms.

Calberg & Kavale note that in the United States, although the inappropriateness of special classes for exceptional children was suggested in the 1930, it was not until the 1960s and 1970s that attention was drawn to children with disabilities. Dunn (1968) advocated the elimination of special classes and schools for more general education classrooms and integrated service-delivery model for students with disabilities, the movement of inclusion is therefore mainly traced back to him. Following Dunn (ibid.) and Reynolds (1989), federal laws focusing on children with disabilities were passed. According to McLeskey and Pacchiano (1994), the Individuals with Disabilities Education Act (IDEA)—previously called The Education for All Handicapped Children Act—enacted in 1975, called for the education (in the least restrictive environment to the maximum extent appropriate) of all children. The law (Public Law 94-142) mandates inclusive education in the general classroom in both public and private institutions. McLeskey and Pacchiano (1994) note further that Section 2 of the law stipulates that it is only when the nature of the severity of the disability is such that education in regular classes with the use of supplementary aids and services cannot be achieved satisfactorily can special classes, separate schooling or removal of disabled children from regular educational environment occur.

Scholars who believe in the inclusionist philosophy in the United States argue that it is the best for all children (Gargiulo, Sluder, & Streitenberger 1997), and that it is beneficial to both disabled and non-disabled students academically, motivationally and affectively (Banerji & Dailey 1995; Salsbury 1991).

According to Giangreco, Dennis, Cloninger, Edelman, & Schattman (1993), many districts in the United States have since 1984 been offering full inclusion to all previously segregated students including those with severe disabilities. In a study titled "Inclusion of students with learning disabilities: Are we making progress" McLesky et al., using expansive and reliable data covering 50 states plus that of the District of Columbia, addresses the dearth of information regarding placement trends for students with learning disabilities and explore the progress made in educating children with disabilities in less restrictive environments. The results show that there was a significant increase in the cumulative placement rate for students with learning disabilities educated in general education classroom between 1988 and 1995. In particular, they noted that the cumulative placement rate for students with learning disabilities educated in the general education classroom for 80% or more of the school day increased by 151% over the six-year period. This increase, they noted, reflected a gain of 614, 000 students. On the other hand, there was a reduction of 18% (140,000 students) in the cumulative placement rate for students with learning disabilities who were educated in resource rooms for 21 to 60% of the school day. The authors also found that students with learning disabilities who were placed in separate school settings decreased by 31%—a reduction of more than 7000 students. The cumulative placement rate for students placed in separate classes increased by 4% (42,000 students).

On the impact of the results on placement practices, it may be noted that there has been an increase (from 45 in 1988/89 to 53 in 194/95) in the number of students with learning disabilities identified. Second, despite the increase in the identification of the students with learning disabilities, there has been no increase in the number placed in highly restrictive separate school or class settings. The number of students with learning disabilities educated in general education classroom has jumped from 9 to 22 whereas the number of those educated in resource settings for 21 to 60% of the school day, decreased from 26 to 21.

Although the results for cumulative placement rate for separate school placements vary little across the U.S. (0-6), there is tremendous variation of inclusive practice regarding other settings. For example, the cumulative placement rate for students educated in separate class settings ranges from 0 to 30, those of resource rooms range from 1 to 51 while the general education classroom range from 4 to 66. They showed that students with learning disabilities in Ohio were twice more likely to be placed in general education classroom than their counterparts in Pennsylvania whereas students with learning disabilities in Pennsylvania were four times as likely to be placed in a restrictive, separate class setting. The comparison of statistics from states with identical policies on inclusion (Ohio and Pennsylvania) also helped to highlight the variation in implementation.

The above results, especially those pointing to a significant increase in the cumulative placement rate for students with learning disabilities educated in general education classroom, are supported by the work of Gargiulo, Sluder, & Streitenberger (1997), Richardson (1998), Stainback and Stainback (1996), and many others.

The fact that there are some states, educators, and parents who either do not support the practice of inclusion, have shown mixed feelings, or are slow in embracing and implementing the inclusion philosophy is supported by the work of Shanker (1995) as well as those of D'alonzo, Giordano and Vanleeuwen's (1997) in New Mexico. Scholars who work on inclusion stated that parents of special need children favor inclusion and most of them are in favor of inclusive settings for their children (Tichenor, Heims, & Piechura-Couture (1998). Concern is also raised by some parents of children without disabilities that less work will be done in school if children with disabilities are included in the general education classroom.

The reaction of teachers toward the inclusionist philosophy is mixed. The work of D'alonzo, Giordano and Vanleeuwen's (1997) in New Mexico on the perceptions by teachers about the benefits and liabilities of inclusion suggest that general education teachers are not optimal disposition toward inclusion by general education teachers. In particular, as much as 81.8% of the respondents felt there would be resistance by teachers. The teachers' responses highlighted the changes needed before they can support inclusion. 83% of the respondents, for example, suggested that personnel who will handle inclusion should be prepared by the universities, 83% said funding procedures should be reorganized, 71.1% called for a change in the curriculum for inclusive classrooms, 70.2% felt that the quality of education would be jeopardized, while 54.8% felt inclusion would not result in the elimination of labeling of students. The above results point to a resistance toward inclusion. Some teachers even think that inclusion could reduce academic progress for the nondisabled, make them lose teacher time and action, and subsequently lead to the acquisition of undesirable behavior from children with disabilities. Others believe that inclusion is 'modified baby sitting' (Wilmore 1994/95). Semmel et al.'s (1991) investigations of attitude toward inclusion seemed to indicate strong teacher opposition to these programs. The responses of teachers in the above investigation suggested that teachers do not believe the instructional needs of students with disabilities can be met in the general education classroom. In effect, despite the overwhelming benefits of inclusion, the results of some researches point to mixed reactions on the part of educators about the benefits of inclusion. However, as Mcleskey and Waldron (1995) rightly posit, most of such investigations were based on teachers being asked hypothetical questions.

In spite of the above concerns, there is enough evidence to support the fact that support for inclusion in the United States has grown significantly. Thus, although researches concerning program effectiveness have produced mixed results regarding the effectiveness of inclusion, there is support for continuing inclusive programs. As noted earlier, McLeskey and Waldron (1995) have indicated that separate classes for students with learning problems have failed to live up to their initial promise and hopes that parents had for them. Furthermore, the Council for Exceptional Children (1993) has also noted that inclusion supports the participation of children regardless of their disabilities in various settings. The works of other scholars like Klinger et al (1998), Marston (1997), bolster the above claims and call on educators to make students with learning disabilities to spend most of the school day in general education classrooms. They also call on educators to deliver most of the services needed by students with learning disabilities to be delivered in the general education classroom settings.

There is no doubt that in the United States the works of Gargiulo, Sluder, & Streitenberger (1997), McLesky and Waldron (1995) and many others point to the immense benefit, especially that of participatory spirit (in the school and home, and in other social domains) by students with learning disabilities who are educated in inclusive settings. Moreover, the studies done on inclusion in the United States point to the fact that in recent years, progress has been made across the U.S. However, as McLeskey rightly points out, there is still insignificant information on why progress has been made on inclusive education and how changes have transpired in some states and failed to materialize in others. In the next section, I discuss the literature on inclusion in Ghana's post-colonial educational system.

INCLUSION IN GHANA'S EDUCATIONAL SYSTEM

The focus of this section is on inclusion in post-independent Ghana paying attention to whether progress has been made and how such progress was made. According to Marfo (1986), before the arrival of Western education, persons with disability were completely excluded from all educational programs.

During colonization, little attention was paid to persons with disabilities and it was not until 1947 that the Presbyterian church opened a school for the visually impaired in Begro and Akropong-Akwapim in Ghana's Eastern Region.

Ghana gained independence from Imperial Britain in 1957. The immediate post-independent educational system paid little attention to the education of people with disabilities and no special attention to inclusion. Marfo notes further that in 1957, an African-American (Rev. Andrew Foster) who was hearing impaired, opened another school for the visually impaired at Christianburg in Accra (Ghana's capital). In 1958, a school for the cripple was built by the Methodist church and this was followed in1964, by a school for the developmentally disabled by Society of Friends Mentally Retarded (Anson 1977).

Avoke & Avoke (1991) note that it was in 1959 that attention was brought to the government of Ghana to the fate of children with disabilities. This led to the calling of parliament into session to pass a bill for the designing of a program for the education and rehabilitation of such children. Parliament, according to the authors, passed a bill making the education for the physically or mentally disabled free and that among other things, making provision for teachers and administrative staff to be trained abroad—especially in the United States, England, and Denmark. The bill passed by parliament mandated collaboration between teachers, parents, the department of education and the department of health in the education of the disabled.

The claim made by Avoke & Avoke (1991) that mainstreaming had not arrived in Ghana in 1992 is wrong and unfounded. As Marfo (1992:113) rightly points out, the General Education Act of 1961 states inter alia "Pupils with special educational needs are included within the general school system, and provision is made for them according to need." It is students whose disabilities are deemed severe and cannot be admitted into the mainstream system who go to the 'special schools'. The biggest problem, however, is that as Ofori-Addo (1995) points out, there are no policies regarding parental involvement in assessment procedures or decision-making regarding children with special needs. Parents are encouraged to send their children to professionals who assess them and decide whether they should join the mainstream educational system; and if so which school the child should go to.

According to the Special Education Policy Act of 1962, at the preschool level, Children with severe mental retardation, visual impairment, and hearing impairment attended Boarding special schools; those with only hearing impairment attended Day special schools; children with severe learning difficulties attend mainstream schools but also get special classes in addition; those with only hearing and/or visual impairment attend regular or mainstream class but have support teaching in such classes. The policy is very strong on integration. In the provision, it is stated that "pupils with physical disabilities are educated in the mainstream" and that "a wide range of support be made available to the regular school—classrooms assistance at preschool level, additional pedagogical support and periodic access to visiting specialists" (P. 114).

A study by Walker, Marfo, Danquah & Aidoo (1986:200-201) provide information to support the above claim and also provide information on specific places where some of the people with specific disabilities were educated. They state *inter alia* that the "blind, deaf, and mentally retarded children are educated and cared for in categorical and segregated settings such as Demonstration School for the Deaf at Mampong-Akwapim. Children with orthopedic problems are educated in mainstream settings." With regard to children with mental disabilities, the authors note that such children are first referred to the Psychiatry Department of the University of Ghana Medical School and the school classifies them into either educable, trainable, and profoundly retarded (see also Danquah, Morson, & Ghanney, 1976; and Ministry of Education, 1974). The educable are placed in mainstream schools whereas the trainable (and some educable) were placed in the Home and School for the Mentally Retarded or the New Horizon School.

Several studies have been done on the advantages of inclusion to the child with disability. A study by Marfo (1992) in the James Town district of the Greater Accra Region, for example, shows several children with speaking and learning difficulties improving in their communicative skills after being taken from special schools and placed in mainstream schools. Such successes, according to Marfo, have led to the formation of Community-based Rehabilitation Programme Advisory Committee and are supported by the University of Ghana in Legon-Accra. The University of Cape Coast in collaboration with the University College of Education (Winneba) have also engaged in a program intended to train peripatetic teachers who offer specialist support for children with disabilities enrolled in mainstream schools.

Odameh (1977) also discusses advantages associated with inclusive education of the deaf in the general education classroom. He notes that the emphasis of the deaf children in these integrated settings was upon speech and lip-reading as a means of communication. He cites a case in Koforidua (Ghana's Eastern Region Capital) where a school that started such an inclusive program in 1975 with 2 students had expanded by 1977 with 14 deaf children in the mainstream school setting. Odameh (ibid.) notes further that during the same period similar successes were scored at Kibi and Adamorabe also in Ghana's Eastern Region. The children involved, according to Odameh, performed better than their counterparts in segregated school in speech communication.

In a study by Dery (1981) on children with speech and communication disabilities, he discovered that pre-schoolers in urban centers enrolled in mainstream educational settings and who had the opportunity to interact with hearing peers, showed great improvement in socialization and oral communication.

Walker et. al. (1986) also point out further that inclusive education in Ghana has been extended beyond preschool and elementary school into high schools and post secondary education. For example, they note that such secondary schools as Wenchi, Navrongo and Okuapeman have admitted deaf and blind students with very encouraging results.

From the above discussion, it is clear that in Ghana, some progress has been made on inclusive education. This measure of success, according to the discussion, has been achieved because of the involvement of the Ministry of Education, the Department of Social Welfare, the Universities providing professional training for the teachers and support staff, and the government of Ghana's willingness to formulate and implement workable policies on inclusive education.

CONCLUSION

From the above discussions, inclusion may be seen as an educational system in which children of school going-age irrespective of their physical or mental status, are brought together and provided with education by professional educators who have the knowledge, willingness, and relevant resources needed for such education to be effective. Inclusion must not lay sole emphasis on students. It must place equal emphasis on the educators, especially preparing the teachers adequately to face the challenge and creating an enabling environment for both teacher and taught. I very strongly share McLeskey & Waldron's (1995:155) concept of what a good inclusive program should have, namely: a program in which students with disabilities make at least as much academic and social progress as they would in a separate classroom; a program in which typical students will make good academic and social progress; provision of support for teachers; and one in which there is normalization (that is, where the rhythm of the day for students with disabilities is as similar as possible to the rhythm of the day for typical students. I believe that if teachers, parents and administrators are willing and able to take the above steps into consideration while developing an inclusive program, a great measure of success will be achieved.

As Marfo (1986) rightly points out, failure or rejection of inclusion shows that such failure or rejection stems form ignorance, fear of the unknown, fear of there being no funds should the program be started, and fear that the educators may not be competent enough to handle problems that may or may not arise. To curtail such fear, it is necessary to create an assurance of support and to initiate programs that will boost the morale and competence to educators.

In the Ghanaian situation, for the inclusive programs to function competently, I will agree with Marfo et.al. (1986) in calling for an improvement in the pre-school and elementary teacher training curricula to include courses on developmental disabilities and special education techniques.

Segregation is baseless and professionally unethical because it is based on unwarranted fear. It is concomitant to encourage teachers, parents, and communities by making available to them the statistics (such as those by McLeskey (1998) in the United States, Marfo (1986) in Ghana, and others) on the successes made by other states or countries that have implemented the inclusive program. People from the successful states or countries may also act as resource personnel in places that are beginning to implement such programs.

In conclusion, it may be argued that there is no doubt that segregating children because of learning disability in not only unfair; it is immoral. Inclusion helps students with learning disabilities and those with no learning disabilities socially, psychologically, and intellectually. With a little education of the educators and policy makers, proper class management by teachers, improving the skills of teachers and removing all 'isms' that hinder inclusion, and goodwill of parents and the public or the community, we can provide equal educational opportunities to all children irrespective of their physical or cognitive disabilities.

REFERENCES

Anson, Y. (1977). History and Development of services for the handicapped in Ghana. Unpublished Manuscript.

Avoke, S.K. & Avoke, M. K. (1992). Development of special education in Ghana. *DISES 2*, 38-39.

Banerji, M. & Dailey, R. (1995). A study of the effects of an inclusion model on students with specific learning disabilities. *Journal of Learning Disabilities, 28* (8), 511-522.

Carlberg, C., & Kavale, K. (1980). The efficacy of special versus regular class placement for exceptional children: A meta-analysis. *The Journal of Special Education, 14* (3), 295-306.

Conderman, G. (1998). How are we practicing inclusion? *Kappa Delta Pi Record, 34(*2), 52-55.

Council for Exceptional Children (1993). Position on inclusion Washington, D.C.

D'alonzo, B.J., Giordano, G. & Vanleeuwen, D.M. (1997) Perceptions by teachers about the benefits and liabilities of inclusion. *Preventing School Failure 42*(1), 4-10.

Danquah, S.A., Morson, J. & Ghanney, E. (1976). Mentally retarded children in hospitals, schools, and homes. *Journal_Psychologie_Africane,* 11(2),199-207.

Dery, S. E. (1981). Childhood deafness and pre-school education in Ghana. *Educafrica,* December (Special Edition).

Dunn, L. M. (1968). Special education for the mildly retarded: Is much of it justifiable? *Exceptional Children, 35*(1), 5–22

Gargiulo, R., Sluder, L., & Streitenberger, D. (1997). Preparing early childhood educators for inclusive programs. A call for professional unification. *Early Childhood Special Education, 25*(2), 137-139.

Giangreco, M., Dennis, R., Cloninger, C., Edelman, S., & Schattman, R. (1993). "I've counted Jon": Transformational experiences of teachers educating students with disabilities. *Exceptional Children, 59* (4), 259-372.

Klinger, J., Vaughn, S., Hughes, M., Schumm, J., & Elbaum, B. (1998). Outcomes for students with and without learning disabilities in inclusive classrooms. *Learning Disabilities research and Practice, 13*(3), 153-161.

Marfo, K. (1986) Confronting Childhood Disability in the developing countries. In K. Marfo, S. Walker, & B. Charles (eds.) Childhood

Disabilities in Developing Countries. Issues in Habilitation and Special Education.pp. 3-27. New York: Preeger Publisher.

Martson, D. (1997). A comparison of inclusion only, pull-out only, and combined service models for students with mild disabilities. *The Journal of Special Education 30*(2), 121-132.

McLeskey, J. & Pacchiano, D. (1994). Mainstreaming students with learning disabilities: Are we making progress? *Exceptional Children, 60*, 508-517

McLesky, J. & Waldron, N. (1995). Inclusive elementary programs: Must they cure students from learning disabilities to be effective? *Phi Delta Kappa, 77*(4), 300-304.

Ministry of Education (1974). *Ghana Education service Bulletin.* Accra: Ghana.

Morgan, A.D. (1991). *New Mexico State Department of Education policy on full inclusion.* State Department of Education. Santa Fe: New Mexico.

Odameh, E. (1977). The Unit School for the Deaf at Koforidua: A report by the headmaster of the school. In K. Marfo, B. J. Aidoo, F. Archer, B. Somuah, & B. Micah (Eds.) *Searchlight On Special Education: A Special Issue Of The Education Searchlight.* Cape Coast: University of Cape Coast Student's Society.

Ofori-Addo, L. (1995). The community-based rehabilitation programme in Ghana. *Department of Social Welfare Report*. Accra: Ghana.

Reynolds, M. (1989). An historical perspective: The delivery of special education to mildly disabled and at-risk students. *Remedial and Special Education, 10*(6), 7-11.

Richardson, R.C. (1998). Inclusion then and now. *KDP Record*. Winter, 49-51.

Sailor, W. (1991). Special education in the restructured school. *Remedial and Special Education, 12*(6), 8-22.

Salisbury, C.L. (1991). Mainstreaming during the early childhood years. *Exceptional Children 58*(2), 146-155.

Semmel, M.I., Abernathy, T.V., Butera, G. & Lesar, S. (1991). Teacher perceptions of the Regular Education Initiative, *Exceptional Children, 58*, 9-24.

Shanker, A. (1995). Full inclusion is neither free nor appropriate. *Educational Leadership, 52*(4), 18-21.

Stainback, S., & Stainback, W. (1996). Inclusion: A Guide for Educators. Baltimore: Paul H. Brookes.

Staub, D. & Peck, C. (1995). What are the outcomes of nondisabled students? *Educational Leadership, 52*(4), 36-40.

Tichenor, M., Heims, B., & piechura-Couture, K. (1998). Putting principles into practice: Parent perceptions of a co-taught inclusive classroom. *Education, 118* (3), 471-477.

Walker, S., Marfo, K., Danquah, A., & Aidoo, B.J. (1986) The Development and Status of Special Education in Ghana. In K. Marfo, S. Walker, & B. Charles (eds.) Childhood Disabilities in Developing Countries. Issues in Habilitation and Special Education. Pp. 191-210. New York: Preeger.

Wilmore, E. (1994/95). When your child is special. *Education*

Chapter 7

Immigrants Share Their Childcare/Preschool Health-Related Experiences in the US

Past Literature

The growth of the foreign-born population in the US has an overall impact on early childhood care practice. Data on immigrants show that the number of immigrants admitted in the US has increases and that they are the fastest growing segment of the US population (Goel et al., 2004). There was an increase of 9.3% for the native population (Malone et al., 2003) while the foreign-born population increased 57%. It is projected that 87% of the population growth between 2005 and 2050 will be driven by immigrants and their US-born children (Passel & Cohn, 2008).

Reviews of the literature on immigrants' health indicate major barriers to acquiring adequate healthcare. For instance, new immigrants in America are largely uninsured, unfamiliar with the U.S. healthcare system, have unique healthcare needs, and do not speak English that would make them function well in the hospital system (Casey, Blewett, and Call 2004; Obeng (2007). The above problems are not easy to solve, since hospitals are hampered in their ability to provide linguistically and culturally appropriate services to these immigrants due to lack of ongoing funding problems (Casey, Blewett, and Call 2004)

Rojas-Guyler, King & Montieth's (2008) work also identify similar problems among immigrants of Mexican descent, not born in the U.S. The authors stated that immigrants of Mexican descent, not born in the U.S. were likely to report having difficulty obtaining health services and lacked knowledge about their health status and illness symptoms. Finally, the authors note that the immigrants were more likely not to utilize available health services.

Obeng's (2007) work on African immigrants also identified similar problems among African immigrants. She noted that African immigrants do not utilize dental healthcare services because of a fear of contracting diseases, financial difficulties, and cultural responsibilities that required them to send money home instead of using the money for their dental health needs.

In view of the problems associated with immigrants' health, it is crucial to examine immigrants health needs and cultural needs while residing in the United States. Given this increase, immigrant children's health will have great impact on the overall health status of the U.S.

Aim of the Study

Given the scholarly work above on immigrants in the U.S., this study qualitatively examined, 50 immigrant parents' childcare/preschool health-related experiences in the U.S.

Methodology

Instrument

The instrument used to collect data for this study was a 7-item questionnaire. The author developed the questionnaire after extensive research and teaching courses on children's health for many years. The survey questions were structured in a way that enabled participants to write their experiences. The instrument consisted of a set of closed- and open-ended questions. The first part consisted of questions that dealt with participant demographics. The second section covered participants' experiences on early childcare education

To ensure the validity of the instrument, the questions were pilot-tested with 10 participants. To ensure sure the wording, level, and nature of the written questions were appropriate for early childcare parents; none of the participants who took part in the pilot study participated in this study.

Participant Selection and Procedure

The study was approved by the Institutional Review Board of Indiana University's Human Subjects Committee. Participants were recruited through *purposeful sampling* (Patton, 1990). 80 research questions were distributed to participants. 50 parents returned the questionnaire, resulting in a response rate of 62.5-%. Some of the parents could not participate because of schedule conflicts. The parents were contacted through e-mails and face-to-face. The study was conducted in 2011/2012. The data were collected by the author as well as graduate students.

Coding and Analysis

The data generated were closely examined by two qualitative researchers. Each of the researchers examined the data separately After examining the data, 2 broad common themes were derived by the coders:

(a) Immigrants favorable experiences in childcare/ preschool in the US
(b) Immigrants Unfavorable experiences

Analysis

Analysis was based on the themes derived from the participants' utterances and their statistical data.

FINDINGS

Parents Demographics

Forty- one participants (82%) identified themselves as having children of preschool aged 3 to 5. Nine (18%) of participants identified themselves as parents of children below the age of two. 75% of the immigrants sent their children to preschools for:

(a) social-emotional growth; and
(b) to prepare them for elementary school.

25% of participants indicated that they sent their children to childcare because of their jobs and schooling.

Favorable Experiences in US Childcare/Preschool

a) Immunization

A participant noted:

> I was glad that children had immunization before they were placed in childcare centers in the US. In my home country children are accepted without looking at their immunization records; this really expose the children to communicable diseases.

b) Sleeping

A participant stated:

> I like the fact that in my child childcare children are allowed to sleep. This is important to me and my child. Sleeping in the afternoon is good for the child.

c) Screening Examinations

A participant expressed:

> My children at Head Start enjoy free periodic dental, ear, and eye screening examinations. I enjoy it because healthcare in the US is very expensive and so this form of assistance is greatly appreciated"

d) Dental Care

A participant noted:

> My child is taught to brush her teeth, wash her hands, etc. Learning this at an early year is great for my child.

Unfavorable Experiences in US Childcare/ Preschools

Although the immigrant parents were enthusiastic about sending their children to preschools the parents complained about:

i) Lack of written policies in childcare/ preschools especially on school attendance
ii) Lack of written policies in some childcare/preschool on allergies.
iii) Lack of education and policies on foods, especially, foreign foods.

The parents noted that the lack of education on foreign foods sometimes leads to teasing and their children not wanting to eat foreign food packed for them.

Some teachers complained about the food that the immigrant parents packed for their children.

Some parents recommended that teachers should be mindful about the comments they make to immigrants, especially, on foreign foods. For example, a parent commented about a remark below given by a teacher: *Is this his lunch-----? Crackers? Or what?*

The parent was unhappy about the teacher's apparent 'disrespect' for the lunch she had packed for her child.

Conclusion and Recommendations

The study recommends that childcare providers should make the following available to immigrant parents through brochures or newsletters:

- When NOT to send their children to school
- When children can get an annual flu shot in the U.S.
- Common childhood illnesses in the U.S.
- Childcare providers should ask parents at the start of the school year whether the parents have any concerns regarding their children's health
- Childcare providers should educate the children and teachers on foreign foods.
- Futures studies should look at health–related polices in childcare/preschools.

REFERENCES

Ahmed, A. T., Quinn, V. P., Caan, B., Sternfeld, B., Haque, R., & Van Den Eeden, S. K. (2009). Generational status and duration of residence predict diabetes prevalence among Latinos: the California men's health study. *BMC Public Health, 9*, 392.

Casey, M. M., Blewett, L. A. & Call, K. T. (2004) Providing health care to Latino immigrants: Community-based efforts in the rural Midwest. *American Journal of Public Health, 94* (10), 1709-1711.

Census 2000 brief. U.S. Census Bureau.

Centers for Disease Control and Prevention (CDC). *1991-2009 High School Youth Risk Behavior Survey Data.* Available at http://apps.nccd.cdc.gov/youthonline. Accessed on 10/19/2011.

Colaizzi, P. (1978). Psychological research as the phenomenologist view it. In *Existential – Phenomenological Alternatives for Psychology*. R. Valle and M. King, (eds.) New York: Oxford University Press, pp. 48-71.

Goel, M. S., McCarthy, E. P., Phillips, R. S., & Wee, C. C. (2004). Obesity among US immigrant subgroups by duration of residence. *JAMA, 292*(23), 2860-2867.

Moran, A., Roux, A. V., Jackson, S. A., Kramer, H., Manolio, T. A., Shrager, Shea, S. (2007). Acculturation isassociated with hypertension in a multiethnic sample. *American Journal of Hypertension*, 20(4), 354-363.

Malone, N., Baluja, K., Costanzo, J., & Davis, C. (2003). *The foreign-born population:* 2000. Census 2000 brief, U.S. Census Bureau.

Passel, J. S., & Cohn, D. (2008). In P.R. Center. (Ed.), *U.S. population projections: 2005-2050.* Washington, DC: Social & Demographic Trends.

Rojas-Guyler, L., King, K. A., & Montieth, B. A. (2008). Health-seeking behaviors among Latinas: Practices and reported difficulties in obtaining health services. *American Journal of Health Education, 39*,25-33

Sokolowski, R. (2000) *Introduction to phenomenology.* Cambridge, UK: Cambridge University Press.

Starks, H. & Trinidad S.B. (2007) Choose your method: A comparison of phenomenology, discourse analysis, and grounded theory. *Qualitative Health Research*, *17*(10),1372-1380.

PART TWO

TEACHING IDEAS

BACKGROUND AND INTRODUCTION

BACKGROUND

Part II of this book is intended to help early childcare educators integrate health education into early childcare settings. This part of the book contains twenty-five activities for children between the ages of two and five. Teachers of young children, or parents, should guide children in doing the various activities. This health education activity book will give teachers and parents the chance to explore various ways that children can be assisted in gaining knowledge about being healthy and skills for healthy living. The health education activities have been connected to *the National Health Education Standards*.

INTRODUCTION

The need for teachers to emphasize health activities in childcare environments cannot be overemphasized. This is because early learning is important for healthy child growth. The habit of washing hands, for instance, reduces disease among children in and out of childcare centers (Kotch et al., 2007). Scholarship on morbidity and mortality rates attributed to injury of children in childcare are unnecessarily high. The high prevalence of accidents among children, along with the attendant need for medical care, illustrates the vital importance of children understanding the contributions that they can make to injury prevention among themselves. Additionally, if any headway is to be made toward reducing childhood injury, then scientific studies about injury causation, management, and prevention among children are warranted.

Children spend much of their day in school, and according to the United States Centers for Disease Control and Prevention (2008), an effective way to prevent violence and injury is for schools to provide better health education. The school environment is the best place to prevent injuries among children.

On the need for making early childhood an important period for studying and imparting health knowledge as well as preventing the spread of disease, scholars have noted that it is during the early years that high-quality care has a positive influence on the cognitive and social development of children (Shlay et al., 2005). In particular, scholars have noted that children who receive good health knowledge and skills at an early age have the propensity to perform well in their academic pursuits. In their work on preventive interventions of diseases, Ells et al. (2005) suggest that during childhood is the most important period for preventive interventions of diseases and risky health behaviors. Rosen et al. (2006) identified preschools as promising venues for enhanced health promotion activities leading to sustained behavioral change. Gupta et al.'s (2005) work also identified childcare centers as places for health promotion.

This Health Education activity book will give teachers and parents the chance to explore various ways that children can learn basic health education and enable them to assist children in gaining the knowledge and skills they need to attain healthy lifestyles. Specifically, this book provides important information and ideas on how health knowledge and skills could be communicated or customized to help children.

The Curriculum Materials Guidelines for Implementing the Curriculum and What the Materials will Help Achieve if Properly Implemented

i) Before talking about food and exercise, teachers/parents should discuss the importance of food with children.
ii) Teachers/parents should stress that our bodies need healthy food in order to grow properly.
iii) Teachers/parents should find appropriate books to read to children before starting the activities.

iv) Please note that this curriculum stems from Vygotsky's (1962) theory of *the Zone of Proximal Development*, which stresses the gap between what children can do by themselves and what they can do with the assistance of more knowledgeable adults. Since the curriculum stems from Vygotsky's (1962) theory of *the Zone of Proximal Development*, it is proposed that teachers or parents first assess the developmental level of children before modifying any materials to suit the children in their setting.

v) Proper implementation of the information in the curriculum will help teachers or parents to use knowledge on a particular health topic to teach concepts like numbers, science, and language development skills to children, and to connect their teaching to the National Health Education Standards.

vi) Proper implementation of these hands-on materials will help children to gain health knowledge and skills that will help them now and in the future.

Instructional Ideas: The examples below are instructional ideas to guide teachers/parents.

PERSONAL HEALTH ACTIVITIES

ACTIVITY 1:
DENTAL HEALTH ACTIVITIES

- ❖ Show children a large picture of children who have normal teeth and a child with tooth decay.
- ❖ Let children locate the differences between the normal teeth and the decayed teeth.
- ❖ Discuss the possible causes of tooth decay with children.
- ❖ Inform children why it is important to brush their teeth twice a day.
- ❖ Invite dental care professionals to your setting to emphasize the need for children to brush their teeth properly.
- ❖ If possible, take children to visit a dental clinic.

STEPS TO INTERGRATE THE ABOVE ACTIVITY INTO OTHER LEARNING AREAS AND WITH THE NATIONAL HEALTH EDUCATION STANDARDS ARE GIVEN BELOW.

AGE	INSTRUCTIONAL ACTIVITIES	INTEGRATION	NATIONAL HEALTH EDUCATION STANDARDS	ASSESSMENT METHODS	REMARKS
3-5 years	❖ Show to children a large picture of children who have normal teeth and a child with tooth decay. ❖ Let children locate the differences between the children with normal teeth and the child with tooth decay. ❖ Ask children about possible causes of the tooth decay. ❖ Inform children about why it is important to brush their teeth twice a day. ❖ Invite a dental care professional to your setting to emphasize the need for children to brush their teeth properly.	**MATHEMATICS** ❖ Children can count the number of teeth in the picture to give them an idea about numbers and counting. **LANGUAGE** ❖ Children can use words to describe the pictures.	**Standard 1:** Core concepts **Standard 7:** Self-management		

Activity 2
Activity on Teeth Brushing

AGE	INSTRUCTIONAL ACTIVITIES	INTEGRATION	NATIONAL HEALTH EDUCATION STANDARDS	ASSESSMENT METHODS	REMARKS
3-5 years	❖ Obtain a denture mold. ❖ Put "dirt" on the denture mold. ❖ Discuss with children why their teeth should be brushed. ❖ Using the denture mold, show children how to brush their teeth. ❖ Ask for a volunteer to try the procedure. ❖ Ask children to practice brushing on the denture mold. ❖ Stress the importance of brushing the teeth twice a day.	LANGUAGE ARTS ❖ Describe the dentures.	**Standard 1:** Core concepts **Standard 7:** Self-management		

ACTIVITY 3
HAND WASHING

Children and caregivers should wash their hands with warm water and soap under the following conditions.

Wash hands:

- ❖ When arriving at school.
- ❖ When returning from the playground.
- ❖ Before cooking activities in the classroom.
- ❖ After cooking activities in the classroom.
- ❖ Prior to drinking.
- ❖ Before and after eating.
- ❖ Before and after brushing one's teeth.
- ❖ Before and after helping a person who is sick.
- ❖ After using the bathroom.
- ❖ Before holding a baby.
- ❖ Before and after changing diapers.
- ❖ After touching doorknobs.
- ❖ After touching railings.
- ❖ After blowing one's nose.
- ❖ After sneezing.
- ❖ After coughing.

THE CENTERS FOR DISEASE CONTROL'S (CDC) (2000) RECOMMENDATIONS FOR HANDWASHING

- ❖ Use warm water.
- ❖ Apply an appropriate quantity of soap.
- ❖ Rub hands together for at least twenty seconds and then rinse hands.
- ❖ Dry hands with a paper towel, and use the paper towel both to turn off the faucet and to open the bathroom door.
- ❖ In the absence of soap and water, it is essential to use ethanol alcohol-based (a minimum 62%) hand sanitizer, preferably in a gel form.

Appropriate Times to Talk about Hand Washing

- ❖ Before going out to the playground.
- ❖ Circle Time, before lunch and snack time.
- ❖ Before naps.

After each activity in the classroom.

ACTIVITY 4
USING THE BATHROOM

Caregivers should conduct activities about the proper use of the bathroom in order for children to avert the possibility of accidentally contacting germs from the improper use of the bathroom. The use of the bathroom should be one of the early activities for childcare providers at the beginning of the semester.

The following are some of the things to talk about often to remind children about the proper use of the bathroom:

- ❖ Do not wait too long to use the bathroom.
- ❖ Always sit properly on the toilet seat.
- ❖ Clean yourself with toilet tissues.
- ❖ Wipe from front to back.
- ❖ Wash your hands using soap and water.
- ❖ Wipe your hands.
- ❖ Remember to turn off the faucet.
- ❖ Remember that the bathroom is not a place to play.
- ❖ Leave the bathroom immediately after you are finished using it.

ACTIVITY 5
COUGHING

CDC provides the following recommendations regarding coughing:

- ❖ It is important to cover one's mouth with a tissue when coughing.
- ❖ Dispose of the tissue in a wastebasket.
- ❖ In the absence of a tissue, cough into one's upper sleeve, not into one's hands.
- ❖ Wash hands with soap and water after coughing.
- ❖ In the absence of soap and water, one should clean hands with alcohol-based hand cleaner.

Activity 6
Activities on Coughing

CDC RECOMMENDATIONS ON COUGHING	INSTRUCTIONAL ACTIVITIES ON COUGHING	INTEGRATION	NATIONAL HEALTH EDUCATION STANDARDS	ASSESSMENT METHODS	REMARKS
❖ Cover mouth with a tissue. ❖ Dispose of the tissue in a wastebasket after use. ❖ In the absence of a tissue, cough into one's upper sleeve. ❖ Do not cough into one's hands. ❖ Wash hands with soap and water after coughing. ❖ In the absence of soap and water, clean hands with alcohol-based hand cleaner.	**Step 1** Demonstrate to children, using a tissue to cover the mouth. **Step 2** Show children the proper way of covering the mouth when coughing. **Step 3** Allow volunteers to demonstrate the procedure. **Step 4** Let interested children practice.	LANGUAGE ARTS Children can use words to describe the procedure.	**Standard 1:** Core concepts **Standard 7:** Self-management		

ACTIVITY 7
NOT PUTTING THINGS IN THE MOUTH

Children should be aware of the dangers of putting the following things in their mouths:

- Coins
- Toys
- Candy
- Large-sized food
- Gum

Caregivers should keep a close watch to ensure that children do not put things in their mouths under the following conditions:

- When children are playing with small items.
- When children are outside playing with pebbles.
- During snack and lunch times, to monitor the size of food that children put in their mouths.

It is important to talk to children about the danger associated with putting certain things in their mouths. Good times to do this include during snack and lunch times, during Circle Time, and before children go to the playground.

ACTIVITY 8
DRINKING WATER FOR GOOD HEALTH

Caregivers should encourage children to drink water in the following ways:

- Showing children where they can get clean drinking water from their setting.
- Providing enough small-size cups appropriate for children at each area where they can drink water.
- Making sure children understand that water is good for their health because it contains no sugar.
- Talking about why people should drink water instead of soda.
- Instructing children about the effect of too much sugar on their dental health.
- Encouraging children to drink water when they are in your care.

ACTIVITY 9
ACTIVITIES ON NUTRITION

Eating Different Kinds of Foods to Improve One's Health

AGE	LEARNING OBJECTIVE (Lesson Behavioral Objective)	MATERIALS AND SUPPLIES NEEDED	INSTRUCTIONAL IDEAS (Strategies with Closure and Transitions)	INTEGRATION	NATIONAL HEALTH EDUCATION STANDARDS	ASSESSMENT METHODS	REMARKS
3 years	To introduce children to different kinds of fruits and vegetables and to encourage them to eat a variety of vegetables served to them.	Pictures of different colors of fruits and vegetables or varieties of flesh fruits and vegetables.	❖ Bring a variety of fruits and vegetables to your setting. ❖ Make sure to include the basic colors of the fruits and vegetables (e.g. red, white, green, blue, black, etc.) ❖ Help children to name the vegetables. ❖ Help children to name the colors. ❖ Let volunteers sort out the fruits and vegetables according to color. ❖ Let children sort the fruits and vegetables according to color. ❖ Let children know the number of minutes that they have before the next activity.	LANGUAGE ARTS Describe of colors. MATHEMATICS Count the different vegetables in each group.	**Standard 1:** Core concepts **Standard 7:** Self-management	Ask children to name some of the fruits and vegetables, especially the ones they like most. Let children identify the color(s) of fruits and vegetables. Ask children to draw the fruits and vegetables. Ask children to group the fruits and vegetables according to taste (e.g., sweet, sour, etc.)	

ACTIVITY 10
INTRODUCING VARIETIES OF FOOD

AGE	LEARNING OBJECTIVE (Lesson Behavioral Objectives)	MATERIALS AND SUPPLIES NEEDED	INSTRUCTIONAL IDEAS	INTEGRATION	NATIONAL HEALTH EDUCATION STANDARDS	ASSESSMENT METHODS	REMARKS
4- to 5-year olds	To introduce children to a variety of foods.	*My Pyramid*, showing a variety of foods from the five food groups. Pictures of fresh foods. Paper plates, glue, and crayons.	Bring different types of food, such as bread, rice, peas, beans, apples, grapes, or milk to your setting. Be sure to include the basic colors: red, white, green, blue, black etc. Ask volunteers to sort out the food according to color. Ask children to sort the foods into groups such as sweets, dairy, fish, etc. This activity can be done in a group or individually.	ART Draw some of the foods. MATHEMATICS Count the different foods in each color group. Putting the foods into a set. LANGUAGE ARTS Use words to describe the foods.	**Standard 1:** Core concepts **Standard 7:** Self-management **Standard 4:** Interpersonal communication	During Circle Time let children talk about the varieties of foods they like most. Allow them to talk freely about why they like particular foods. Let children draw the foods that they like the most. Teachers can, by using *My Pyramid* guidelines, teach children why they should or should not eat certain foods that they like in excess.	

ACTIVITY 11
NUTRITION ACTIVITIES FOR THREE-YEAR-OLDS

Note: This activity is for three-year-olds

AGE	INSTRUCTIONAL IDEAS	INTEGRATION	NATIONAL HEALTH EDUCATION STANDARDS	REMARKS
3 years	Create two charts: one containing healthy foods and one containing unhealthy foods. Include corresponding pictures of the food and let children place them on the chart. Ask volunteers to try out the procedure. Allow children to try the activity This activity can be done individually or in groups.	LANGUAGE ARTS Describe, using color, the foods used. MATHEMATICS Collect foods into a set.	**Standard 1:** Core concepts **Standard 7:** Self-management	

Activity 12
Placing Favorite Foods on Paper Plates

Age	LEARNING OBJECTIVE (Lesson Behavioral Objectives)	MATERIALS AND SUPPLIES NEEDED	INSTRUCTIONAL IDEAS	INTEGRATION	NATIONAL HEALTH STANDARDS	ASSESSMENT METHODS	REMARKS
3 years	To assist and encourage children to eat a variety of foods.	Pictures of a variety of vegetables, fruits, meat, fish, milk, bread, etc.	❖ Bring in a variety of pictures of foods. ❖ Let children choose pictures of foods they like most and place them on paper plates. ❖ Ask volunteers to talk about what they have placed on their plates. ❖ Stress the importance of eating from all food groups.	LANGUAGE ARTS Describe the food on their plates. MATHEMATICS Collect favorite foods into a set.	Standard 4: Interpersonal communication	Children and caregivers discuss the food in each child's plate.	

Activity 13
Healthy Foods and Unhealthy Foods

AGE	LEARNING OBJECTIVE (Lesson Behavioral Objectives)	MATERIALS AND SUPPLIES NEEDED	INSTRUCTIONAL IDEAS	INTEGRATION	NATIONAL HEALTH STANDARDS	ASSESSMENT METHODS	REMARKS
4- to 5-year olds	To teach children the foods that they should eat the most.	Crayons Papers Pictures of both healthy foods and unhealthy foods.	Create two charts: one containing healthy foods and one with unhealthy foods. Discuss with children why some of the foods are healthy and others are not. Find other pictures of healthy foods and ask children to match the healthy foods to the group of healthy foods already discussed. Stress to children that the foods matched in the healthy group should be eaten the most. This activity can be done individually or in groups.	LANGUAGE ARTS Describe of colors. MATHEMATICS Collect food into a set.	**Standard 1:** Core concepts **Standard 7:** Self-management	Check to make sure children have matched food items correctly into their corresponding categories.	

Activity 14
Using Stories to Encourage Children to Eat Healthy

AGE	LEARNING OBJECTIVE (Lesson Behavioral Objectives)	MATERIALS AND SUPPLIES NEEDED	INSTRUCTIONAL IDEAS	INTEGRATION	NATIONAL HEALTH STANDARDS	ASSESSMENT METHODS	REMARKS
3 years	To encourage children to make good choices about what to eat for optimal growth when food is served to them.	Materials for your story.	❖ Devise a story that is appropriate for the child's or children's situation. ❖ If children are not eating their vegetables, create a short story about why it is important for them to eat vegetables. ❖ If possible, look for children's books that talk about the importance of eating vegetables to read to children. ❖ Look for the vegetables that appear in your story and bring them in for your lesson. ❖ During the course of the story, pause and ask children choose the vegetables that appear.	MATHEMATICS Picture-matching	**Standard 5**: Decision-making **Standard 7:** Self-management	Make sure children choose the fruits or vegetables appropriate to the story.	

Appropriate Times to Talk about Food

- During cooking time in the classroom.
- During snack and lunch time.
- Before and after working in a vegetable garden during the summer.

Make sure the above lessons are used to encourage children to eat different kinds of food for optimal development. Always stress in your lessons the importance of eating healthy foods (e.g., eating fruits and vegetables).

ACTIVITY 15
PHYSICAL ACTIVITY TO ENHANCE HEALTH

Caregivers should take the following into consideration in order to reduce the occurrence of Injuries during physical activity:

- Supervise children closely during playtime.
- Set feasible rules with children and enforce the rules while they play.
- Caution children against running unnecessarily during playtime.
- Caution children against pushing each other.
- Model appropriate behavior for children so that they will not engage in any behavior that will lead to injuries.
- Give children developmentally appropriate activities that make use of fine and gross motor skills during playtime.
- Make sure there is enough room for gross motor skills activities such as walking, running, skipping, and riding toy cars on your playground.
- Make sure children do not shove, bump into, or step on each other.
- Make sure children do not fall.
- Make sure children do not trip.
- Make sure children are not too crowded in a particular play area.
- Make sure children do not fight on the playground.
- Make sure children do not throw objects at each other.

Note: Injuries are the leading cause of death among children in industrialized countries.

AGE	LEARNING OBJECTIVE (Lesson Behavioral Objectives)	MATERIALS AND SUPPLIES NEEDED	INSTRUCTIONAL IDEAS	INTEGRATION	NATIONAL HEALTH STANDARDS	ASSESSMENT METHODS	REMARKS
3-5 years	To provide a safe environment for children to engage in physical activity for the improvement of their health.		❖ Ask children to name the equipment that they know on the playground. ❖ Show pictures of all of the playground equipment to the children. ❖ Ask volunteers to name playground equipment shown to them during Circle Time. ❖ Inform children of the equipment that they do not know. ❖ Take children to the playground and make sure they know the names of the equipment and how to use them. ❖ Encourage children to share equipment when necessary.	LANGUAGE ARTS Describe the equipment, using color. MATHEMATICS Place equipment into sets according to color.	**Standard 1:** Core concepts **Standard 7:** Self-management **Standard 5:** Decision-making	Ask children to name the equipment, and demonstrate to you how to use and share the equipment.	

ACTIVITY 16
PLAYGROUND SAFETY

Familiarize children with playground equipment in order to ensure that they understand how to use it and consequently ensure safety as children enjoy the physical activities.

This activity should be done at the beginning of each school year and should be continued until the teacher is certain that the children understand and are comfortable with all equipment on the playground.

Concerning injury prevention, *familiarizing children with playground equipment* at the beginning of the year helps prevent injuries among children. Teaching children the names of all the equipment and demonstrating how to use it at the beginning of the school year will help the children gain knowledge on the proper use of equipment on the playground.

Appropriate Times to Talk about Playground Safety

- During Circle Time.
- Before going to the playground.
- On the playground.

ACTIVITY 17
MAKING RULES ABOUT PLAYGROUND EQUIPMENT

AGE	LEARNING OBJECTIVE (Lesson Behavioral Objectives)	MATERIALS AND SUPPLIES NEEDED	INSTRUCTIONAL IDEAS	INTEGRATION	NATIONAL HEALTH STANDARDS	ASSESSMENT METHODS	REMARKS
3-5 years	To help children stay safe on the playground.		❖ Discuss the use of playground equipment. ❖ Come up with rules for the use of equipment. ❖ Ask volunteers to name the rules. ❖ Ask children to repeat rules. ❖ Repeat the rules during Circle Time. This activity should be done in a group.	LANGUAGE ARTS Describe the rules.	**Standard 1:** Core concepts **Standard 7:** Self-management	Ask children to remind the teacher and the classmates of the rules about playground safety.	

ACTIVITY 18

RIDING A BICYCLE: RIDING FOR FUN AND IMPROVING YOUR HEALTH

AGE	LEARNING OBJECTIVE (Lesson Behavioral Objectives)	MATERIALS AND SUPPLIES NEEDED	INSTRUCTIONAL IDEAS	INTEGRATION	NATIONAL HEALTH STANDARDS	ASSESSMENT METHODS	REMARKS
3-5 years	To encourage children to ride a bicycle and to be safe when riding bicycles.		❖ Talk about the importance of riding a bicycle. ❖ Discuss possible answers. ❖ Ask children to suggest different ways to exercise in order to stay healthy. ❖ Stress the importance of wearing a helmet while riding a bicycle. ❖ Talk to children about safe places in the school where children can ride their bicycles. ❖ Discuss the rules that children should follow at home when riding a bicycle: (a) Stay at the location agreed upon with parents	LANGUAGE ART Describe their bicycles, using color. ART Draw bicycles and tricycles.	**Standard 1:** Core concepts **Standard 7:** Self-management **Standard 4:** Decision-making	Let children try riding their bicycles, being mindful of the rules.	

			(b) Go with an adult who can assist with traffic (c) Always ride facing oncoming traffic (d) Remember to sit properly on the seat while riding a bicycle. ❖ This activity should be repeated to make sure children are familiar with the guidelines for riding a bicycle.				

Appropriate Times to Talk about Bicycle Safety

❖ During Circle Time: If bicycle safety is discussed during normal Circle Time, try to find a book about bicycles to read to children before going to the playground.

Activity 19

Encouraging Physical Activity in the Classroom

AGE	LEARNING OBJECTIVE (Lesson Behavioral Objectives)	MATERIALS AND SUPPLIES NEEDED	INSTRUCTIONAL IDEAS	INTEGRATION	NATIONAL HEALTH STANDARDS	ASSESSMENT METHODS	REMARKS
3-5 years	To help children stay active inside the classroom.		❖ Before Circle Time, and with the supervision of the teacher, let children do physical activity before they sit down for circle time. ❖ An example of an activity is shown below: ❖ Select three children and ask them to take 10 steps forward, turn around and then take ten steps backwards before they sit down for Circle Time. ❖ Encourage all children to be active before they sit down to do any activity. ❖ Teachers should always take active part in all physical activities. ❖ Teachers should be role models for children during physical activity lessons.	LANGUAGE ART Describe their bicycles, using color. ART Draw bicycles and tricycles.	**Standard 1:** Core concepts **Standard 7:** Self-management **Standard 4:** Decision-making	Make sure children are encouraged to participate in the activity.	

ACTIVITY 20
CHOOSING A FAVORITE PHYSICAL ACTIVITY TO PERFORM IN ORDER TO HELP CHILDREN GET THEIR DAILY RECOMMENDED PHYSICAL ACTIVITY

Group 1

With the supervision of the teacher, let a child choose one of the following activities to do for 20 minutes:

- Ride a bicycle.
- Swing.
- Play on monkey bars.
- Play basketball.
- Play football.
- Play soccer.
- Play baseball.

Group 2

Below is an idea to help children get 5 to 10 minutes of their recommended physical activity. Choose one of the following activities to do with children.

In-class activities:

- Ask children to sit and stand before Circle Time. Do this several times.
- Ask children to jog for a few minutes before sitting down for Circle Time.

Group 3

Below is an idea to help children get 25 to 30 minutes of their recommended 60 minutes physical activity. Teachers may choose one of the following activities that are appropriate for their setting:

- Walk with children to find out what they like about nature.
- Gardening.

The above activities can be integrated into topics in Science, Mathematics, Art (drawing), and Language Arts.

ACTIVITY 21
FIRE SAFETY

Discuss with children what can cause fire at school and in the house:

- Stove.
- Electrical outlet.
- Matches.
- Lighter.
- Heaters.

AGE	LEARNING OBJECTIVE (Lesson Behavioral Objectives)	MATERIALS AND SUPPLIES NEEDED	INSTRUCTIONAL IDEAS	INTEGRATION	NATIONAL HEALTH STANDARDS	ASSESSMENT METHODS	REMARKS
3-5 years	To teach children about fire safety.		❖ Discuss with children why they should not touch the following: stove, electrical outlet, matches, lighter, heater. ❖ Brainstorm for ideas about why children should not touch the above things; e.g., burning results in hospital admission or missing school. ❖ Ask volunteers to name some of the things that can burn them. This activity should be done in a group.	LANGUAGE ARTS Describe why children should not touch things that can cause fire without adult supervision.	**Standard 1:** Core concepts **Standard 7:** Self-management	Ask children to remind the teacher and the classmates of the rules about playground safety.	

ACTIVITY 22

TALKING ABOUT NOT TOUCHING DANGEROUS THINGS: SCISSOR SAFETY

AGE	LEARNING OBJECTIVE (Lesson Behavioral Objectives)	MATERIALS AND SUPPLIES NEEDED	INSTRUCTIONAL IDEAS	INTEGRATION	NATIONAL HEALTH STANDARDS	ASSESSMENT METHODS	REMARKS
4-5 years	To teach children about how to use scissors		❖ Explain to children why they should not run with scissors and that they could hurt themselves or someone else. ❖ Describe how to use a pair of scissors safely. ❖ Show children how to hold the scissors. ❖ Let children practice using scissors. ❖ Tell children that if they see any of their classmates, siblings, or friends running with scissors, they should stop them and show them the correct way to handle the scissors. ❖ Tell children NEVER to run while holding a pair of scissors.	ART Draw scissors Cut different shapes of scissors and let children color them	**Standard 7:** Self-management **Standard 5:** Decision-making	Make sure children understand that they should not run with scissors.	

Appropriate Times to Talk about Scissors Safety

- ❖ Before art and craft lesson.
- ❖ How to integrate these into traditional subjects:
  - -Art (cut out pieces of materials that focus on a given topic and glue them together).
  - -Math (cut out shapes or fruits, vegetables, pictures of milk or different types of cereal, and add them together).
  - -English (cut out alphabets letters).
  - -Science (cut out animals and different kinds of fish and identify them)

ACTIVITY 23
GUN SAFETY

LEARNING OBJECTIVE (Lesson Behavioral Objectives)	MATERIALS AND SUPPLIES NEEDED	INSTRUCTIONAL IDEAS	INTEGRATION	NATIONAL HEALTH STANDARDS	ASSESSMENT METHODS	REMARKS
To teach children about gun safety.		❖ Ask children whether they have a toy gun. ❖ Ask children when and where they use their toy guns. ❖ Tell children not to touch any gun that does not belong to them. ❖ Teach children to always tell an adult if they see a gun. ❖ Teach children NEVER to play with any gun that is not theirs	ART Draw toy guns.	**Standard 7:** Self-management **Standard 5:** Decision-making	Make sure children are encouraged not to touch guns that do not belong to them, including family members.	

ACTIVITY 24
MEDICINE SAFETY

AGE	LEARNING OBJECTIVE (Lesson Behavioral Objectives)	MATERIALS AND SUPPLIES NEEDED	INSTRUCTIONAL IDEAS	INTEGRATION	NATIONAL HEALTH STANDARDS	ASSESSMENT METHODS	REMARKS
4-5 years	To teach children about medicine safety.		❖ Discuss with children when they should take medicine. ❖ Tell children not to touch any medicine even if it belongs to them. ❖ Teach children to always tell an adult if they see any medicine sitting out. ❖ Tell children NEVER to play with medicine.	ART Children draw any medicine they have ever seen	**Standard 7:** Self-management **Standard 5:** Decision-making	Make sure children understand that they should not touch any medicine.	

ACTIVITY 25
KNIFE SAFETY

AGE	LEARNING OBJECTIVE (Lesson Behavioral Objectives)	MATERIALS AND SUPPLIES NEEDED	INSTRUCTIONAL IDEAS	INTEGRATION	NATIONAL HEALTH STANDARDS	ASSESSMENT METHODS	REMARKS
3-5 years	To teach children about knife safety.		❖ Discuss with children the times when their parents use knives. ❖ Tell children not to touch any knives. ❖ Tell children to always tell an adult if they see any knives at school or at home. ❖ Tell children NEVER to play with knives.	LANGUAGE-ART Adults assisting children to describe why they should not touch a knife	**Standard 7:** Self-management **Standard 5:** Decision-making	Make sure children understand that they should not touch any knives.	

REFERENCES

Centers for Disease Control and Prevention (2008). Injury and Violence. http://www.cdc.gov/HealthyYouth/injury/index.htm

Ells, L. J., Campbell, K., Lidstone, J., Kelly, S., Lang, R., & Summerbell, C. (2005). Prevention of childhood obesity. *Best Practice & Research Clinical Endocrinology & Metabolism, 19*(3), 441-454.

Gupta, R. S., Shuman, S., Taveras, E. M., Kulldorf, M., & Finkelstein, J. A. (2005). Opportunities for health promotion education in child care. *Pediatrics, 116*(4), 499-505.

Kotch, J. B., Isbell, P., Weber, D. J., Nguyen, V., Savage, E., Gunn, E., Skinner, M., Fowlkes, S., Virk, J., & Allen, J. (2007). Hand-washing and diapering equipment reduces disease among children in out-of-home child care centers. *Pediatrics, 120*(1), 29-36.

Rosen, L., Manor, O., Engelhard, D., Rosen, B., Peleg, H., Meir, M., & Zucker, D. (2006). Can hand-washing intervention make a difference? Results from a randomized controlled trial in Jerusalem preschools. *Preventive Medicine, 42*(1), 27-32.

Shlay, A. B., Tran, H., Weinraub, M., & Harmon, M. (2005). Teasing apart the child care conundrum: A factorial survey analysis of perceptions of child care quality, fair market price and willingness to pay by low-income, African American parents. *Early Childhood Research Quarterly, 20*(4), 393-416.

Vygotsky LS (19962). *Thought and Language*. Cambridge, MA: MIT Press.

ENCOURAGING HEALTHY EATING

INTRODUCTION

A difficult situation is often created for preschool teachers when children refuse to eat during lunch or snack time. Such a situation often emanates from the teachers' love for, and concern about, the welfare of the children they care for, as well as the professional, social, and legal issues associated with care-giving. Teacher educators, preschool teachers, nutritionists, pediatricians, as well as parents often attempt various creative means of solving the problem of poor eating, sometimes, to no avail. The problem of children's poor eating is exacerbated when it comes to the consumption of fruits, and more especially, vegetables given the fact that children often find these vegetables and fruits unattractive and without the kind of taste they are used to finding in candies and other sweetened foods and non-alcoholic beverages.

A way out of a situation in which children are not motivated to eat certain kinds of food is to use stories that will enlighten the children about the importance of those kinds of food and the necessity of making them part of their diet. This is because children love stories. Stories also act as a channel through which important, and often-delicate facts, may be communicated to children (Cook, 2001; Obeng, 2006).

Through stories, preschool teachers are able to share their time, attention, and emotional involvement with the children cognizant of the fact that appropriate use of stories draws adult preschool teachers to the children (van Maanen, 1991). Stories, thus, constitute a necessary foundation for early childhood education because of educators' ability to use them to teach the essential rules and strategies for living, for survival, for coping with challenging situations, and for solving day-to-day problems (Cook, 2001).

OBJECTIVES

Given the importance of stories in Early Childhood Education, and in view of some children's resistance to food offered them, the purpose of this paper is to provide ideas on creating stories on healthy eating and assess the impact of the stories on children's eating behavior

MATERIALS AND SUPPLIES NEEDED FOR THE LESSON

(a) Papers and different types of crayons.
(b) Samples of real vegetables, fruits, or any food talked about in the story.
(c) Glue
(d) Pictures that contain the foods about which the stories will be told.
(e) Paper plates.

TARGET AUDIENCE

The target audience is children and preschool teachers.

GUIDELINES FOR CREATING AND TELLING STORIES ABOUT HEALTHY EATING

The following are general guidelines for creating and telling stories about healthy eating to children in order to encourage those with poor eating habits to eat well. The guidelines were arrived at based on the author's many years of teaching in preschools and also on her experience as a teacher educator (professor and supervisor of preschool/early childhood teachers).

Guidelines

These guidelines are based on Grice's (1975) communication maxims that enjoin communicators to aim for an effective interactional cooperation. The original Gricean maxims are: quality (truthfulness), quantity (exactness or saying just enough), manner (simplicity and avoidance of obscurity), and relevance (speaking only relevantly). The guidelines given here extend the Gricean maxims and adapt them to the preschool setting to ensure maximum and effective communication between teachers and children in preschools. They are stated as follows:

1. Be simple: Do not use jargon or technical terminology that will be incomprehensible to the children. Avoid obscure language. Use names, persons, and foods known to the children. A picture is worth more than a thousand words so, if possible, have a picture of a real food item on hand.
2. Avoid exaggeration: Although stories are by nature fictional, avoid saying things that you cannot justify or things that are plainly wrong.
3. Be relevant: Do not tell stories that are not relevant to the issue or problem at stake. Using simple language, stress the importance of eating the food, fruit, or vegetable about which the story is told.
4. Be concise: Do not tell too long or too short a story. An unusually long story invites boredom. On the other hand, a story that is overly short may not be informative enough and may therefore be ineffective in communicating the intended ideas.
5. Observe the child's reaction: After finishing the story, observe the child's reaction to the story. If the reaction is that of enthusiasm and acceptance, stress parts of the story they liked most during snack and lunchtime to remind them to make good use of the story in making good choices in eating their meals. On the other hand, if the reaction is that of disinterest and/or rejection do not react negatively. Rather, change the topic and come back to it some other time/day. Whatever the result/reaction, it is essential to give the child an assurance and support.

Procedure

Besides the above general guidelines, it is incumbent upon preschool teachers to observe, and where necessary, adhere to the following important guiding principles when imparting knowledge about healthy eating on children:

i. Before telling healthy-eating related stories to any group of children, ensure that you have available, all the necessary educational resources (e.g., pictures, paper, crayons, etc.) that will aid effective communication.
ii. If you anticipate having the children do some work during the story-telling time, make sure you distribute the required resources before telling the story.
iii. Tell the story.
iv. During the telling of the story, you may show the children samples of real vegetables, fruit, or any food talked about in the story.
v. Ask the children to draw or talk about any event or episode of the story that interests them.
vi. Repeat the story.
vii. Use stories creatively to engage children. This could be done by creating expressive and performance strategies that call on children to dramatize, sing, paint, or draw aspect of the story

Guidelines for Classroom Activities

The children may be asked to do the following activities:

(a) Dramatize the story
(b) Sing parts of the story
(c) Draw some of the food they like best
(d) Select pictures that contain the foods about which the stories are told.
(e) Glue the pictures on paper plates.
(f) Share personal experiences about the foods.

Evaluation Questions and Measures for the Story-Telling

Objectives	Evaluation questions	Evaluation outcomes
1. To Create and tell stories about healthy eating to preschoolers.	Were you able to create and tell the story?	Actual number of stories created and told.
2. Make available opportunities for the children to create their own stories.	Did the story-time provide opportunities to the preschool children to create their own stories?	Actual number of stories created by the preschool children.
3. To provide preschoolers with the opportunity to change eating habits	Did the story influence the preschoolers' ideas about eating fruits and vegetables?	Actual number of the preschool children who were influenced by the story. This could be done by observing children at lunch or snack time and by talking to parents. Also, activities done by children such as drawing some of the foods mentioned in the story or picking up pictures containing foods about which the stories were told.
4. Provide opportunities for the preschoolers to learn about fruits and vegetables	Were opportunities provided for the preschoolers to learn about fruits and vegetables?	Number of opportunities provided for the preschoolers to learn about fruits and vegetables.
5. Provide opportunities for the preschoolers to share experiences acquired during the story-telling time.	Were opportunities provided for the preschoolers to share their experiences about eating vegetables and fruits?	Number of times that the preschoolers shared their experiences.

Impact

It is anticipated that the stories will have considerable impact on the teachers and children. In particular, it is anticipated that there will be:

1. A surge in interest and consumption of fruits and vegetables by the preschoolers
2. A significant enrichment in the teaching style of preschool teachers.
3. A considerable improvement in the learning and lifestyle of the preschoolers.
4. Boost preschoolers' overall interest in and knowledge about healthy eating.
5. Enhance teachers' overall competence in health education.

Caution

Teachers must know that there are several strategies for influencing children's behavior and that storytelling is one of such strategies. It is important for the preschool teacher to know the multiplicity of classroom situations, the uniqueness of each situation, and different communication strategy each situation calls for. Taking the overall classroom context into consideration has a considerable impact on the effectiveness of the teaching methodology that is employed. Knowing what story to tell is important; even more important is knowing how, when, and where to tell it as well as what age group to tell it.

Conclusion

It is essential for preschool teachers to create stories that emphasize the importance of eating well. Specifically, such stories must be self-explanatory. Also such stories could be created to focus on foods that children are picky about.

In sum, it is important to emphasize the fact that because of children's interest in stories and their unique listening skills, preschool teachers can capitalize on such interest to teach a great deal of health-related information through stories.

Appendix (Sample Story)

Children's Story on Healthy Eating: A Lesson on Foods that Make you Strong

Mr. Fruits

Once upon a time there was a man called Mr. Fruits. Mr. Fruits lived in a small town called "Eat-An-Orange" and he told this beautiful story to the children. The story was about eating foods that help to make people strong. Mr. Fruit's story went like this:

"Once there were ten boys and girls who were four and five year olds. The name of their school was Fruit and Vegetable Childcare. They were very good friends and liked to eat different foods, but they did not like to eat their fruits and vegetables. However, a little boy named Sam and a little girl named Pam loved to eat fruits and vegetables. Pam and Sam always ate their fruits and vegetables at lunchtime.

Because Sam and Pam ate a lot of fruits and vegetables, they were very strong. They did not always have to go to the doctor to get shots. Sam and Pam were so strong that whenever they went on the swings they could swing high. They were also brave because they were never scared of falling off the swings. They had a firm grip on things.

However, the other children who ate foods that did not strengthen their muscles were not as strong as Sam and Pam. They were always sad because they wanted to be strong too.

So they asked their caregiver, 'How can we be strong like Sam and Pam?' The caregiver said, 'Well, if you eat apples, bananas, oranges, peaches, pineapples, carrots, tomatoes, and peas, you will be healthy and strong too.' One child, called Josh said, 'Ok, I will eat all of my fruits and vegetables for lunch everyday.' Josh also became strong and very happy. Soon the other children began eating their fruits and vegetables and they also became healthy and strong. They could also swing high on the swings like Sam and Pam.

They were so happy. This made their parents and their teacher happy too! You know what, children, an apple a day keeps the doctor away."

REFERENCES

Cook, W. J. (2001). Create and tell a story: help young children who have psychological difficulties. *Young Children 56*(1), 67-70.

Grice P. (1975). Logic and conversation. D. Davidson, & G. Harman (Eds.) *The Logic of Grammar.* Encino, CA: Dickenson. Pp. 64-75.

Obeng, C.S. (2006). Strategies for teaching stories to young children. *Canadian Children 31*(1), 22-28.

van Maanen, M. (1991). *The Tact of Teaching*. Albany, NY: State University of New York.

SOCIO-CULTURAL SENSITIVITIES IN THE EARLY CARE CLASSROOM: MANAGING EMOTIONAL RELATED PROBLEMS IN CULTURALLY DIVERSE EARLY CARE SETTINGS

As humans there is often the tendency for us to make numerous assumptions about what is or is not the norm. It is often all too easy to see certain unfamiliar behavioral patterns as being uncouth, morally degenerative, anti-social or unacceptable and hence needing immediate abolishment. And, despite the fact that we speak of our society and our communities as being diverse, the tendency has been for us to assume like-mindedness, similarity in culture, an in some cases, similarity in behavioral patterns and belief systems.

Much as it is important to emphasize what binds humans together, it is also important to recognize the fact that there are important differences, especially, with respect to culture and behavior. Being in one and the same environment or setting must however not be seen as having identical behavior, emotional state of mind, or culture. Emotional or behavioral patterns deemed appropriate in one culture may be seen as a taboo in another culture. Such opposite spectra can cause major problems in childcare domains. It is important to note that people from different cultures react to identical situations differently. Culture may determine how one reacts to a problem and the extent to which such a reaction influences one's health. It is for this reason that childcare providers must take children's cultural background differences into consideration when caring for them. Ignoring the cultural differences can result in one's inability to efficiently manage the children's mental and emotional needs.

The following will be useful when working with children from diverse backgrounds:

- Learn (from the parents of students) some cultural differences that may trigger emotional problems in the child. There are basic non-verbal and/or extra-linguistic features which you may consider as normal in mainstream American culture but which can very easily trigger discomfort or emotional problems in settings where there are children with multicultural backgrounds.
- Here are a few examples from other cultures:

Looking Someone Straight in the Eye

In some Asian, Caribbean, and African cultures looking someone straight in eye while talking with them is considered rude and disrespectful toward the person. Forcing a child from any of the above cultures to look at you in the eye may create fear and panic in the child.

Showing the Sole of Your Foot

In some Asian societies (such as Nepal), showing the sole of your foot is an indication of disrespect toward the person that you are showing it to. In as much as possible, avoid showing the sole of your foot to them. Alternatively, you can inform the children and their parents that it is alright to do that in the United States.

Use of the Thumb

In some African cultures raising your thumb is an insult to one's mother. This, of course, is not the case in American society where it signifies a job well done. Giving a mere thumb up could therefore stimulate discomfort in some children of African origin.

Giving Somebody Something with the Left Hand

In some non-Western cultures giving someone anything with your left hand indicates disrespect for the person because the left hand is used in doing acts that are considered unclean. In some cases, giving a child from such cultures anything with the left hand may create a sense of dislike and anger since they may see the teacher as not respecting them. Again, you may initially not use this gesture and then gradually tell the children that it is alright to do that in American society.

The Volume/Loudness of One's Voice

In some non-Western societies children are expected to speak with a low volume when speaking with an adult (including teachers). Speaking with a loud voice is seen as rude. It is also considered normal for an adult to use a high volume when talking with a child since that suggests seriousness and authority. Not using the right volume could create a problem. For example, a reprimand may be ignored or not seen as serious if it is done in a low volume.

General Guidelines for Helping Children in Diverse Classrooms to Deal with Emotional Problems

- Avoid immediate and/or spontaneous attempts at 'reforming' an individual's emotional problems without looking at their cultural backgrounds. It is all too easy to see other people's experiences, cultures, and values as being less important than yours and hence resorting to mainstream disciplinary strategies.
- Avoid belittling or labeling behavioral patterns resulting from students' unique cultural backgrounds. This could, in an extreme cases, lead to exclusionism, xenophobia, and outright anger.
- Let children know how to take turns in all activities. Stepping in or interrupting someone can sometimes initiate severe emotional problems in some children. Some children may see such an act as an attempt to stop them from contributing in a discussion or even an attempt at shaming them.

- It is important to bear in mind that behavioral patterns may be adopted and shed according to the requirements of different social or cultural situations. In particular, it is important for you to recognize the fact that the boundaries of students' emotional and mental outlooks expand and contract in response to new settings including new teacher-student or student-student interactional settings, in different groups, or in a changed stimuli. Not paying attention to the above-mentioned social, cultural, and interactional domains may result in one form of emotional problem or the other.
- Furthermore, it is important to recognize the fact that children's various personalities and behavioral patterns derive from several sources including nationality, ethnicity, social class, community, gender, and culture.
- To be successful in helping children to manage or control their emotional problems, you must manage your own emotional problems. Do not forget that children always learn from you.
- Do not ignore problems that arise from emotion. For instance, if a child comes to you with a problem that arises from anger, it is important to put yourself in the same camera angle as the child and communicate with her in a non-threatening manner. By putting yourself in the same "shoes" as the child, the child sees you as a person who is concerned about him/her and is willing to help solve it. This strategy works perfectly in most care-giving environments.
- Avoid being judgmental when it comes to solving problems that arise from emotion because being judgmental can trigger further emotional problems in some children.
- In a conflict situation, allowing the children engaged in the conflict to freely express themselves works better than shoving the problem beneath or under the rug.
- The good old saying, *patience is a virtue*, is a golden rule in dealing with children's emotional problems. It is important to be patient while, at the same time, being careful in the selection of words and expressions that help to ease or eliminate such problems. Always end conflict resolutions by letting the children know you appreciate their involvement in solving the problem. Congratulate them for the good job done.

- Finally, you must recognize your limitations. Never shun the services of professional counselors when dealing with children-related emotional problems.

INDEX

D

E

F

G

H

I

O

P

Q

R

S

T

U

V

W

X

Y